STUDY GUIDE FOR

Safe Maternity and Pediatric Nursing Care

Luanne Linnard-Palmer, EdD, MSN, RN, CPN

Nursing Professor

Dominican University of California

San Rafael, California

Gloria Haile Coats, MSN, RN, FNP

Nursing Professor

Modesto Junior College

Modesto, California

F.A. Davis Company • Philadelphia

F. A. Davis Company
1915 Arch Street
Philadelphia, PA 19103
www.fadavis.com

Printed in the United States of America

Last digit indicates print number: 10 9 8 7 6 5 4 3 2 1

Publisher, Nursing: Terri Wood Allen
Manager of Project and eProject Management: Catherine H. Carroll
Senior Content Project Manager: Christine M. Abshire
Art and Design Manager: Carolyn O'Brien

As new scientific information becomes available through basic and clinical research, recommended treatments and drug therapies undergo changes. The author(s) and publisher have done everything possible to make this book accurate, up to date, and in accord with accepted standards at the time of publication. The author(s), editors, and publisher are not responsible for errors or omissions or for consequences from application of the book, and make no warranty, expressed or implied, in regard to the contents of the book. Any practice described in this book should be applied by the reader in accordance with professional standards of care used in regard to the unique circumstances that may apply in each situation. The reader is advised always to check product information (package inserts) for changes and new information regarding dose and contraindications before administering any drug. Caution is especially urged when using new or infrequently ordered drugs.

ISBN 978-0-8036-2495-5

Reviewers

Lori Airth, RN
Practical Nursing Instructor
Northern Lakes College
Valleyview, Alberta, Canada

Mary T. Amundson, RN, MSN
Practical Nursing Faculty
Northland Community and Technical College
East Grand Forks, Minnesota

Janice Ankenmann-Hill, RN, MSN,
    CCRN, FNP-C
Professor and Program Director, Vocational and Associate
    Degree Nursing
Napa Valley College
Napa, California

Darlene Baker, RN, MSN
Director of Health Career Programs
Green Country Technology Center
Okmulgee, Oklahoma

Holli Benge, RN, MSN
Professor/Department Chair
Tyler Junior College
Tyler, Texas

Melanie Benington, RN, MSN
Practical Nursing Training Specialist
Cuyahoga Community College
Cleveland, Ohio

Kristie A. Berkstresser, PhD, RN, CNE, BC
Associate Professor of Nursing
HACC, Central Pennsylvania's Community College
Lancaster, Pennsylvania

Christi Blair, RN, MSN
Nursing Faculty
Holmes Community College
Goodman, Mississippi

Jammie Blankenship, RN, MSN
Practical Nursing Instructor
Kiamichi Technology Centers
Hugo, Oklahoma

Cheryl Bruno-Mofu, RN, ADN
Instructor of Vocational Nursing and Allied Health
Palo Verde College
Blythe, California

Karen Clark, RN, MSN
Instructor of Nursing/Full Time Faculty
Lehigh Carbon Community College
Schnecksville, Pennsylvania

April Cline, RN, CNE, PhD
Practical Nurse Educator, Instructor
Isothermal Community College
Spindale, North Carolina

Michelle Crum, RN, BSN, EJD
Practical Nursing Program Director
Ozarks Technical Community College
Springfield, Missouri

Mary Davis, RN, MSN
Nursing Instructor
Wiregrass Georgia Technical College
Valdosta, Georgia

Natalie Deleonardis, MSN, RN
Coordinator of the North Campus Outreach Practical
    Nursing Program
Pennsylvania College of Technology
Wellsboro, Pennsylvania

Sharon Demers, RN, BN, CAE
Instructor
Assiniboine Community College
Winnipeg, Manitoba, Canada

Sally Flesch, RN, BSN, MA, EdS, PhD
Professor, Coordinator, Practical Nursing Program
Black Hawk College
Moline, Illinois

Tina Forrester, MSN, RN
Practical Nursing Instructor
Bladen Community College
Dublin, North Carolina

Louise S. Frantz, RN, BSN, MHA, Ed
Coordinator Practical Nursing Program
Penn State Berks
Reading, Pennsylvania

Nadra Gibson, RN, BSN
IDNEP
Academy of Medical & Health Science
Pueblo, Colorado

Alice Gilbert, RN, BSN
Director, Instructor
Ukiah Adult School Vocational Nursing Program
Ukiah, California

Linda Griffis, RN
Lead Instructor
Practical Nursing Program
Pearl River Community College
Poplarville, Mississippi

Marie Hedgpeth, RN, MSN, MHA
Practical Nursing Faculty
Robeson Community College
Lumberton, North Carolina

Catherine Krahn Horton, RN, MSN
Nursing Instructor
Madison Area Technical College
Fort Atkinson, Wisconsin

Melody Jaymes, RN, MSN
Practical Nursing Instructor
Huntingdon County Career and Technology Center
Mill Creek, Pennsylvania

Valerie Jenkins, RN, BSN
Quarter 3 Coordinator
Galen College of Nursing
San Antonio, Texas

Kathy A. Johnson, RN, BSN
Practical Nursing Instructor
Greater Lowell Technical School
Tyngsboro, Massachusetts

Robin Kern, RN, MSN
Program Chair, Practical Nursing
Moultrie Technical College
Moultrie, Georgia

Lori A. Koehler, FNP-C, MSN, RN, CEN
Faculty
Northampton Community College
Bethlehem, Pennsylvania

Kelly Kidd, RN, BScN, MN
Professor, Coordinator Practical Nursing Program
Algonquin College
Pembroke, Ontario, Canada

Tracy Lohstroh, MSN
Nursing Faculty/Department Chair for Allied Health
Shawnee Community College
Ullin, Illinois

Nancy Lyons, RN, BSN
Instructor, Coordinator LPN Program
Holy Name Medical Center School of Practical Nursing
Teaneck, New Jersey

Patricia C. Martin, RN, MS
Chair of Nursing, Calmar Campus
Northeast Iowa Community College
Calmar, Iowa

Kathleen J. Maschka, RN, MSN
Nursing Faculty
Minnesota State College – Southeast Technical
Winona, Minnesota

Lynda Matthews, RN, BSN
Coordinator of Practical Nursing Program
Texas County Technical College
Houston, Missouri

Kim McCombs, RN, MSN
Assistant Professor
Black Hawk College
Moline, Illinois

Carolyn McCormick, RN, MSN, CNE
Director Practical Nursing Program
Cape Fear Community College
Wilmington, North Carolina

Judy Melton, RN, MSN
Assistant Director Practical Nurse Education
McDowell Technical Community College
Marion, North Carolina

Barbara Michalski, RN, MSN
Practical Nursing Instructor
Tulsa Technology Center
Tulsa, Oklahoma

Marybeth Millan, BSN, RNC, CCE
Nurse Educator
Ocean City Vocational Technical School
Toms River, New Jersey

Nancy Morris, RN, MSN, Ed
Director/Instructor of Practical Nursing Program
North Georgia Technical College
Toccoa, Georgia

Tracy Moshier, RN, MSN, CCE
Nursing Instructor
Lake Superior College
Duluth, Minnesota

JoAnne M. Pearce, MS, RN
Assistant Professor
Idaho State University
Pocatello, Idaho

Tammy Pehrson, RN, MS
Practical Nursing Program Manager
College of Southern Idaho
Twin Falls, Idaho

Patrice Pierce, RN, MSN
Director of Nursing Program
Central Georgia Technical College
Milledgeville, Georgia

Cheryl Lynn Puckett, MSN, RNC-OB
Associate Professor
Bluegrass Community and Technical College, Danville
    Campus
Danville, Kentucky

Heather (Thomas) Reardon, RN, MS
Associate Professor
College of Southern Idaho
Twin Falls, Idaho

Dana Reece, RN, MSN/Ed
Professor of Nursing
Horry Georgetown Technical College
Georgetown, South Carolina

LuAnn J. Reicks, RN-BC, BSN, MSN
Professor/Practical Nurse Coordinator
Iowa Central Community College
Fort Dodge, Iowa

Ellen Santos, RN, MSN, CNE
Director of Practical Nursing
Assabet Valley Regional Technical School
Marlborough, Massachusetts

Anna Schmidt, RN, MA, PHN
Dean of Health Sciences
Hennepin Technical College
Brooklyn Park, Minnesota

Glynda Renee Sherill, RN, MS
Practical Nursing Instructor
Indian Capital Technology Center
Tahlequah, Oklahoma

Anne Simko, RN, BSN, MS
LPN Department Head
Eli Whitney Technical School
Hamden, Connecticut

Carolyn Slade, AAS
Practical Nursing Instructor
Wiregrass Georgia Technical College
Fitzgerald, Georgia

Rox Ann Sparks, RN, MSN, MICN,
    LNC, ENPC
Assistant Director Vocational Nursing
Merced College – Dr. Lakkireaddy Allied Health Division
Merced, California

Kelly Stone, RN, BSN
PN Program Coordinator
University of Arkansas Community College at Batesville
Batesville, Arkansas

Miranda Stover, RN, BS, MSN
Assistant Professor of Practical Nursing
Iowa Lakes Community College
Emmetsburg, Iowa

Serena Strain, RN, MSN
Nurse Faculty, Lead Instructor
Forsyth Technical Community College
Winston Salem, North Carolina

Sandy Wallace, RN, MS, BA
Professor of Nursing
Kansas City Kansas Community College
Kansas City, Kansas

Resa Yount, RN, BSN
Practical Nursing Senior Instructor
Tennessee College of Applied Technology
Morristown, Tennessee

Note to the Student

The *Study Guide for Safe Maternity and Pediatric Nursing Care* has been written by the authors to accompany the textbook, *Safe Maternity and Pediatric Nursing Care.* Each chapter contains a variety of exercises that will assist you to learn and apply the chapter content. In our own classroom settings, we have found these types of exercises to be beneficial for our students studying maternity and pediatrics. We hope you will use this *Study Guide*, as well as the great resources on the Davis*Plus* Web site, to assist you in studying for exams. Mastering the maternity and pediatric content will prepare you to pass the NCLEX® exam and to provide safe and effective nursing care for maternity and pediatric patients. *Study Guide* answers are posted on the instructor's Davis*Plus* Web site. Ask your instructor about accessing answers.

Each chapter has a variety of exercises that may include:

• NCLEX-style review questions
• True or false questions
• Matching exercises
• Short answer questions
• Fill-in-the-blank questions
• Essay questions
• Crossword puzzle
• Concept maps
• Table completion exercises
• Labeling exercises

Suggestions for Success!

As educators, we have found the following suggestions to be helpful for students to be successful in nursing school:

• *Read all of the assigned reading.* Reading before class will make it easier to understand the instructor's lectures and classroom activities.

• *Complete every exercise in the Study Guide.* This will reinforce the textbook and lecture and improve your retention of the material.
• *Utilize the online resources that supplement the textbook content on the Davis*Plus *Web site.* There are additional exercises available for each chapter.
• *Join a study group.* When you are a member of a study group that meets regularly and works through the class material, you will be better prepared. Take turns reviewing course content, talk through information that is more difficult to understand, and support each other.
• *Don't get behind.* There is a large amount of outside class reading and studying that you must do. "Cramming" material right before an exam rarely leads to understanding the material and scoring excellent test grades.
• *Limiting your outside obligations can be helpful.* Balancing family, school, and work can be difficult. Scheduling your time can only be done by you. Be wise in your choices.

We hope you find this *Study Guide* useful.
Luanne Linnard-Palmer and Gloria Haile Coats

Contents

unit ONE

Introduction to Maternity and Pediatric Nursing

Healthy People 2020 and Initiatives for Healthy Families

Name: _Giavanna Martin_

Date: _____

Course: _VN130_

Instructor: _____

LEARN TO C.U.S.
SHORT ANSWER QUESTION

You are caring for a family who brings their newborn infant into the Public Health Department clinic asking for bottles of formula. The mother is tearful and says that although she has tried to nurse the infant, she is not producing milk. This is the young family's first baby. You take the baby's height, weight, and head circumference and find that the height and head circumference is within the 50th percentile for an infant of almost 4 weeks of age, but the weight has not changed since the reported birth weight.

Using the Learn to C.U.S. method of communicating, how might you express your concerns to your team members?

C: _____

U: _____

S: _____

TEAM WORKS

Matching Exercise

Match the Leading Health Indicator with the family-related example that affects mothers, babies, children, and teenagers:

B 1. Access to health care
E 2. Preventive services
C 3. Air quality
A 4. Injury and violence
D 5. Maternal, infant, and child health
F 6. Mental health

A. Homicide and suicide
B. All families should have insurance coverage and a consistent primary care provider
C. Clean land, air, water; free from lead and allergens
D. Child abuse and neglect
E. Immunizations
F. Adolescent depression

SAFETY *STAT!*

TRUE OR FALSE QUESTIONS

1. *F* The original landmark document created by the Surgeon General was created in 1991 to address the status of health of the American people. This influential document had the purpose of setting goals for the improvement of health of all people.

2. *F* Communication disorders currently addressed by the *Healthy People 2020* child section include autism spectrum disorder, hearing loss, and the need for more aggressive antibiotic treatment for otitis media.

SAFETY *STAT!*

REVIEW QUESTIONS

1. Who is responsible for monitoring progress toward the objectives set by *Healthy People 2020*?
   1. Nonprofit local organizations
   (2) Epidemiologists
   3. Nurse executives
   4. State-run hospital collectives

2. Some of the *Healthy People 2020* topics pertain to populations at large, such as children and teens. Which of the following are examples of *Healthy People 2020* topics for children? (*select all that apply*)
   (1.) Nutrition
   (2.) Mental health
   3. Hypertension prevention
   (4) Injury prevention

CULTURAL CONSIDERATIONS

Draw an illustration of your family tree with the names of at least three generations and the health-care concerns, diseases, and age of death for each member. Start by drawing a tree with the various branches being members of your family.

TEAM WORKS
TRUE OR FALSE QUESTION

__T__ Data exist showing progress toward the goals up to the year 2011. Progress is divided into the categories of target met, improvement occurring, worsening, or no change/unable to tell.

TEAM WORKS
FILL-IN-THE-BLANK QUESTION

Healthy People 2020 is an important document for all health-care professionals to review and understand.

Healthy People 2020 aligns with the projection that a ___larger___, ___older___, and ___more___ ___diverse___ United States population is on the horizon.

TEAM WORKS
SHORT ANSWER QUESTIONS

1. The overall goals for *Healthy People 2020* are based on three overall outcomes. List the three outcomes based on these goals:

   1. ___↑ life expectancy___
   2. ___improve quality of life___
   3. ___Eliminate health disparities___

2. Many organizations have been involved in working toward the achievement of the proposed objectives of the *Healthy People* initiative. These organizations include federal agencies and non-federal agencies. List four of these organizations with at least one being a non-federal agency.

   1. _____
   2. _____
   3. _____
   4. _____

SAFETY *STAT!*
SHORT ANSWER QUESTION

The *Healthy People 2020* objective related to breastfeeding includes three topics. List the three topics:

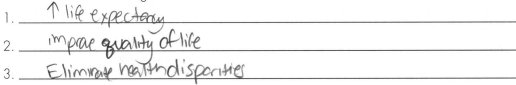

1. ___↑ the % of employers who have worksite lactation programs___
2. ___↓ % of breastfed newborns who recieve formula within first 2 days of life___
3. ___↑ % of live births in facilities that recommend care for lactating mothers___

unit TWO

Pregnancy and the Family

Introduction to Maternity Nursing

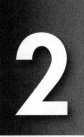

Name: _____

Date: _____

Course: _____

Instructor: _____

REVIEW QUESTIONS

1. What triggered the onset of family-centered care in the maternity units of hospitals?
   1. The founding of maternity hospitals
   2. The introduction of the Lamaze and Bradley methods for labor
   3. The use of scopolamine to control pain in labor
   4. The introduction of visiting nurses

2. The most common causes of death in childbirth prior to the 20th century were: (*select all that apply*)
   1. Infection
   2. Herbs taken for pain control
   3. Hemorrhage
   4. Hypertension disorders
   5. Malpresentation of the fetus

3. A patient is struggling with making a decision regarding the health care of her premature newborn. Ethically, the nurse should: (*select all that apply*)
   1. Give the patient advice on the right decision to make.
   2. Be careful not to impose personal values on the patient.
   3. Provide the patient with information to make a decision.
   4. Ask another patient with a premature baby to talk to her.

4. A nurse has been assigned to a patient in labor and delivery. The patient states that she is homeless and did not receive any prenatal care. The nurse that is assigned to this patient completes an admission assessment and assists the patient to bathe while waiting for the assigned physician to arrive. The nurse is demonstrating the ethical principles of:
   1. Trust and autonomy
   2. Nonmaleficence and honesty
   3. Justice and standards of care
   4. Justice and beneficence

5. A new graduate nurse is assigned to the postpartum unit. A postoperative Cesarean patient is having complications. The physician has ordered a nasogastric tube to be inserted. The nurse has only inserted one nasogastric tube as a student with her instructor's assistance. The correct action for the nurse would be to:
1. Review the procedure in the hospital procedure manual.
2. Tell the physician that she has never inserted a nasogastric tube.
3. Ask a coworker how to insert a nasogastric tube.
4. Try to remember the correct steps while at the bedside.

TRUE OR FALSE QUESTIONS

1. _F_ Nursing students can provide better care for a postpartum patients if they have children.

2. _T_ Physicians took control over the labor and birthing process during the early 20th century.

3. _F_ A maternity nurse practitioner can deliver babies in the hospital.

4. _T_ Standards of care describe the level of performance expected of a nurse.

5. _F_ A nurse can perform duties outside the scope of practice if directed to do so by a physician.

TABLE COMPLETION

List the five roles of nurses and their education requirements and general services they provide.

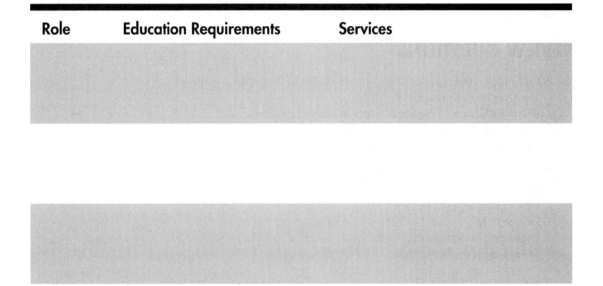

Role	Education Requirements	Services

POST-CONFERENCE QUESTIONS

Short Answer Questions

1. What persons or factors influenced your decision to become a nurse?

_____

_____

_____

_____

_____

2. Are you considering continuing education in order to become an advanced practice nurse? If so, why or why not?

_____

_____

_____

_____

_____

LEARN TO C.U.S.
SHORT ANSWER QUESTION

In the labor and delivery unit, a student nurse accompanies a doctor into the patient's room. The patient tested positive to group B streptococcus and was supposed to be receiving an IV infusion of an antibiotic through the piggyback route. The previous nurse had brought the medication into the room and attached it to the patient's primary line but had neglected to set the infusion pump and turn it on. The doctor looks at the student nurse and says, "Get those IV antibiotics started, now! It's here, all you have to do is turn it on." The student nurse knows that IV medication infusions are not part of her scope of practice. The student nurse answers the doctor using the C.U.S. method of communication.

C: _____

U: _____

S: _____

MATCHING EXERCISE

Match the example of a nursing action with the ethical term.

D 1. The nurse questions the doctor about a dose of medication that seems too much for a patient.

C 2. A patient decides not to have a blood transfusion.

A 3. A nurse offers pain medication to a postoperative Cesarean patient.

B 4. All patients are treated the same.

A. Beneficence
B. Justice
C. Autonomy
D. Nonmaleficence

CASE STUDY
SHORT ANSWER QUESTION

Janette gave birth a few hours ago. Her baby had breathing problems at birth, and he is in the neonatal intensive care unit. Janette wants to breastfeed her baby, but the nurses say that he is too sick to breastfeed right now. Janette is very upset. She has strong feelings about breastfeeding and is disappointed that the doctors and nurses will not let her try to feed him. How can the nurse promote autonomy for this patient in this situation?

_____
_____
_____
_____
_____

Concerned
Uncomfortable
Safety

FILL-IN-THE-BLANK QUESTIONS

1. Nursing care based on current scientific knowledge is called _evidence based knowledge_.

2. _Ethics_ are moral principles that guide behavior.

3. The legal outline of what a nurse can do according to the laws of the state is called the _scope of practice_.

4. Nurses became patient _advocates_ when they assisted women with presenting birth plans to their physicians.

5. If a nurse observes an unsafe practice, the usual method for reporting up the organizational ladder in a hospital is called the _C.U.S._.

Human Reproduction and Fetal Development

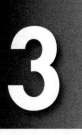

Name: _____

Date: _____

Course: _____

Instructor: _____

REVIEW QUESTIONS

1. A woman comes to the clinic for information. She plans to start trying to get pregnant in 3 months. What advice by the nurse is appropriate?
   1. "Lose as much weight as possible so you can gain weight with the pregnancy."
   2. "You may take any medications you have been taking regularly."
   3. "Decrease alcohol consumption."
   4. "Be cautious of environmental hazards that could harm a developing fetus."

2. A pregnant woman at 12 weeks' gestation smokes "a few" cigarettes a day. She wants to stop smoking. She asks if she can use the nicotine patch safely. The best advice from the nurse is:
   1. "Yes, that's better than smoking."
   2. "No, it causes vasoconstriction and is not recommended for pregnancy."
   3. "I would recommend the nicotine gum."
   4. "It's too late to stop smoking now; the damage is done."

3. The primary functions of the testes are:
   1. Fertilization and testosterone production
   2. Fertilization and sexual arousal
   3. Testosterone production and sperm production
   4. Testosterone production and sexual arousal

4. The internal organs of female reproduction are: *(select all that apply)*
   1. Labia majora
   2. Ovaries
   3. Uterus
   4. Vagina
   5. Mons pubis

5. The primary functions of the ovaries are:
   1. Ovulation and hormone production
   2. Ovulation and sexual response
   3. Ovulation and fertilization
   4. Ovulation and pelvic support

FILL-IN-THE-BLANK QUESTIONS

Fetal Circulation

Fetal circulation begins when oxygenated blood from the placenta enters the fetus through the ___umbilical___ ___vein___. The oxygenated blood bypasses the liver through the ___ductus___ ___venosus___ and combines with deoxygenated blood in the inferior vena cava. Blood then rejoins deoxygenated blood from the superior vena cava and empties into the ___right atrium___. Pressure is greater in the right atrium than the left atrium, so most blood will move through the ___foramen___ ___ovale___. A small amount of blood does travel from the right atrium to the right ventricle into the pulmonary system, but most bypasses the pulmonary arteries and moves directly into the aorta through the ___ductus___ ___arteriosus___ and out to the rest of the body. Deoxygenated blood returns to the ___placenta___ through the ___umbilical___ ___arteries___.

MATCHING EXERCISES

Match the following terms with their correct description.

___D___ 1. Amniotic fluid
___G___ 2. Amniotic membrane
___B___ 3. Cervix
___H___ 4. Teratogen
___E___ 5. Embryo
___A___ 6. Endometrium
___F___ 7. Dizygotic twins
___I___ 8. Placenta
___J___ 9. Umbilical cord
___C___ 10. Wharton's jelly

A. Mucous membrane that lines the cavity of the uterus
B. The lower portion of the cervix that projects into the vagina
C. A gelatinous substance that provides support and protection for the vessels inside the umbilical cord
D. Provides buoyancy, movement, and protection for the fetus
E. The stage of development between fertilized ovum and fetus
F. Fraternal twins developing from two separate sperm and ova
G. A thin membrane that surrounds the fetus and amniotic fluid
H. Any substance that can cause a birth defect
I. Provides the fetus with nourishment and oxygen
J. Joins the fetus to the placenta

CASE STUDY
PATIENT TEACHING GUIDELINES

The nurse in the gynecology office has an appointment with Felicia and Roberto Lopez. Felicia is 38 years old, and she wants to begin a family. She has a family history of twins. They have many questions about conception, the chance of having twins, and the safety of medications. Answer the following questions for Felicia and Roberto.

1. "Is it possible that I could have twins?"
2. "I always thought that fertilization happened in my uterus. Is that true?"
   in fallopian tube

3. "What can I do to prepare for a healthy pregnancy?"
4. "What about my asthma medication? Should I stop taking it?"
5. "Is there anything I could do to prevent birth defects?"

TABLE COMPLETION

Placental Hormones

Using the information in your textbook, complete the following table.

Hormone	Function
Progesterone	• regulates condition of the inner lining (endometrium) completes the development • calms & quiets the uterine muscle to allow for successful implantation
Estrogen	↑ female characteristics (enlargement of breasts, endometrium, regulation of menstrual) • stimulates growth of the myometrium & improves blood flow to the placenta & fetus • prepares for breastfeeding
Human chorionic gonadotropin	• supports the development of the embryo • used to determine pregnancy either by urine or blood test
Human placental lactogen	• assists w/ milk preparation & metabolism during pregnancy
Relaxin	• works w/ progesterone • causes relaxation of pelvic ligaments to aid in birthing

CASE STUDY: SAFETY *STAT!*

Jennifer, age 22, is a college student. She came to the Emergency Department with physical complaints of nasal congestion, cough, sinus pressure, and a headache. She is diagnosed with a sinus infection. What questions should the nurse ask before the antibiotics are prescribed?

CULTURAL CONSIDERATIONS

Interview a pregnant woman from a different culture or ethnic group. Ask her about any cultural taboos regarding pregnancy or childbirth that have been expressed to her during her pregnancy. Share your findings at clinical postconference.

CASE STUDY: TEAM WORKS

Carla, age 30, wants to start a family. She is 5'2" tall and weighs 250 pounds. She is concerned about weight gain in pregnancy and her health-care provider is encouraging her to lose weight before becoming pregnant. She states, "I want to lose weight, but I need help." What suggestions should the nurse give Carla regarding weight loss? What team members should be included in Carla's plan to lose weight?

THERAPEUTIC COMMUNICATION

Using therapeutic communication techniques and the ACOG Five A's, prepare a discussion with a pregnant woman who smokes. The American College of Obstetricians and Gynecologists (ACOG, 2011) suggests that the nurse use the Five A's model to address smoking in pregnancy.

1. Ask about tobacco use.
2. Advise her to quit.
3. Assess about willingness to make an attempt to quit.
4. Assist in her quit attempt.
5. Arrange for follow-up.

CONCEPTUAL CORNERSTONE

The concept of reproduction is a foundational concept in the biological sciences. This chapter begins the discussion of this concept of human reproduction. The scope of this concept ranges from normal reproductive health to problems associated with reproduction. Discuss the normal menstrual cycle leading to ovulation and possible pregnancy.

Physical and Psychological Changes of Pregnancy

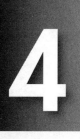

Name: _____

Date: _____

Course: _____

Instructor: _____

SHORT ANSWER QUESTIONS

Diagnosis of Pregnancy

List the signs and symptoms commonly associated with the three categories of a pregnancy diagnosis.

Presumptive signs of pregnancy

1. Nausea & Vomiting
2. Fatigue
3. Urinary frequency
4. breast enlargement & tenderness
5. Amenorrhea
6. Quickening

Probable signs of pregnancy

1. Goodell's sign - softening of the cervix
2. Ballottement - feeling the fetus floating away from the body
3. Chadwick's sign - bluish purple coloration of the vaginal mucosa & cervix
4. Hegar's sign - softening of the lower uterine segment
5. + Pregnancy test

Positive signs of pregnancy

1. Fetal heart heard by Doppler
2. Fetus movement
3. Ultrasound

MATCHING EXERCISE

_L_ 1. Amenorrhea
_F_ 2. Anemia
_H_ 3. Ballottement
_D_ 4. Chadwick's sign
_A_ 5. Dysuria
_I_ 6. Goodell's sign
_K_ 7. Hegar's sign
_E_ 8. Hemorrhoids
_J_ 9. Kegel exercise
_C_ 10. Melasma
_B_ 11. Quickening
_G_ 12. Striae gravidarum

A. Painful or difficult urination
B. Awareness of the movement of the fetus
C. Brown facial skin discoloration
D. A deep blue color of the vagina and cervix
E. Enlarged veins in the anus and rectal area
F. A reduction in circulating red blood cells
G. Stretch marks
H. A diagnostic pregnancy maneuver in which the fetal part rebounds when touched by an examiner's finger
I. Softening of the cervix
J. An exercise for strengthening the vaginal and perineal muscles
K. Softening of the lower uterine segment
L. Absence of menstruation

REVIEW QUESTIONS

1. The pregnant patient is expected to be aware of fetal movement by approximately how many weeks of gestation?
   1. 6 to 8 weeks
   2. 10 to 12 weeks
   3. 14 to 16 weeks
   4. 18 to 20 weeks

2. At her prenatal visit at 34 weeks' gestation, a patient confides that she has noticed an increase in vaginal discharge. The nurse's response should be to:
   1. Advise her to wash with non-irritating soap three times a day.
   2. Advise her to abstain from sexual intercourse.
   3. Ask her if the discharge is irritating or itchy.
   4. Ask her to buy an over-the-counter medication for treatment.

3. A patient complains that the iron supplement she is taking causes constipation. The best response by the nurse is: (_select all that apply_)
   1. Increase fluids.
   2. Increase exercise.
   3. Stop taking the medication.
   4. Take the medication with a glass of milk.
   5. Increase fiber in the diet.

4. A woman in her second trimester of pregnancy is discussing her relationship with her mother and how happy she is that her mother is "excited about becoming a grandmother." According to Rubin (1984) and Mercer (1995), this patient is completing which task of pregnancy?
   1. Ensuring safe passage for herself and her fetus
   2. Seeking acceptance of the child by others
   3. Learning to give of self and to accept herself as mother to an infant
   4. Committing herself to the child

5. Tara, age 17, at 32 weeks' gestation, is very concerned about the dark brown areas on her face that have occurred during the pregnancy. The appropriate response by the nurse is: (_select all that apply_)
   1. "The hyperpigmentation usually disappears after childbirth."
   2. "The skin is never the same after pregnancy."
   3. "Using sunscreen may reduce the severity."
   4. "You need a referral to a dermatologist."
   5. "It is caused by increased levels of hormones of pregnancy."

6. A pregnant patient has been prescribed an iron supplement by her health-care provider. What information should be provided by the nurse?
   1. "This supplement will replace your prenatal vitamins."
   2. "Take this supplement with a meal."
   3. "This supplement is better absorbed with a liquid containing vitamin C."
   4. "Take this supplement with the prenatal vitamins."

7. The nurse is examining a woman who is at 20 weeks' gestation. The nurse would expect the fundus to be:
   1. At the level of the symphysis pubis
   2. Midway between the symphysis pubis and the umbilicus
   3. At the level of the umbilicus
   4. Above the umbilicus

8. What should the nurse teach a pregnant patient regarding the changes in her cardiovascular system during pregnancy?
   1. She will have fewer red blood cells.
   2. She may become dizzy if she lies on her back.
   3. She may bleed more easily due to increased platelets.
   4. She may notice a decrease in her pulse rate.

9. A woman arrives for her prenatal appointment. She is at 36 weeks' gestation. Which discomfort of pregnancy does the nurse expect?
   1. Nausea
   2. Tender breasts
   3. Headache
   4. Backache

10. Which finding is considered a probable sign of pregnancy?
    1. Chadwick's sign
    2. Urinary frequency
    3. Tender breasts
    4. Fetal heart rate heard with a Doppler

NURSING CARE PLAN: Teamwork

Alisa is 22 years old. She lives in a small apartment in a large city with her husband, Keith. She is at 8 weeks' gestation and is experiencing nausea. She states, "I work as a model. I thought we would have a family someday, but this pregnancy happened sooner than I planned. I am so nauseous; I haven't eaten in 2 days. When do you think I will start showing? It will be hard for me to work when that happens."

Prepare nursing diagnoses appropriate for this situation and include referrals to appropriate health team members in the interventions.

💬 THERAPEUTIC COMMUNICATION

Margo, age 39, has accompanied her 19-year-old daughter to her first prenatal appointment. Margo mentions, "I don't think I want to be a grandmother." What therapeutic responses would be appropriate in this situation?

CULTURAL CONSIDERATIONS

Bahula is of Indian descent. She is 24 years old and 12 weeks pregnant with her first child. She lives with her husband and his family. She states that she feels good and is not sure that she really needs prenatal care. "My mother and mother-in-law give me advice about pregnancy. They didn't need a midwife until they delivered their babies." What response by the nurse is appropriate in this situation?

PATIENT TEACHING GUIDELINES: BREAST CARE DURING PREGNANCY

Prepare a mini teaching plan about breast care during pregnancy.

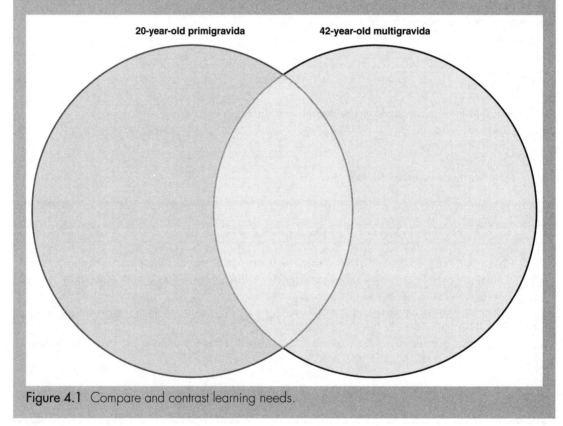

CONCEPTUAL CORNERSTONE

Each pregnant woman's experience is unique. Patient teaching plans must be developed according to the individual patient's needs. Compare and contrast the possible learning needs of a 20-year-old primigravida and a 42-year-old who is pregnant for the fourth time.

20-year-old primigravida   42-year-old multigravida

Figure 4.1 Compare and contrast learning needs.

POST-CONFERENCE ACTIVITIES

1. Discuss the importance of early prenatal care in the prevention of complications and promotion of a healthy and safe pregnancy.
2. During the clinical experience, interview a pregnant woman or a postpartum patient from a different culture. Students should evaluate cultural responses of the woman and her family to pregnancy and use of the health-care system.
3. Invite a woman who is pregnant or has given birth to twins or other multiples to discuss her pregnancy discomforts and experiences with the students.
4. Search the nursing literature for articles related to pregnancy discomforts and effective nursing measures. Summarize the key points of one article during the post-clinical conference time.

Antepartal Nursing Assessment

5

Name: _____

Date: _____

Course: _____

Instructor: _____

SHORT ANSWER QUESTIONS

An initial health history is important to planning patient-centered care. Provide three questions to ask the patient for each category of the initial health history.

Personal Information

1. _____
2. _____
3. _____

Family History

1. _____
2. _____
3. _____

Cultural, Religious, and Spiritual History

1. _____
2. _____
3. _____

Current Medical History

1. _____
2. _____
3. _____

Gynecological and Obstetrical History

1. _____
2. _____
3. _____

Current Medical History

1. _____
2. _____
3. _____

Current Pregnancy

1. _____
2. _____
3. _____

FILL-IN-THE-BLANK QUESTIONS

Provide the correct GTPAL for each patient.

1. Margaret is pregnant for the fourth time. She has three living children all born at 40 weeks gestation and living. G:4 T:3 P:0 A:0 L3

2. Jennifer is pregnant for the fifth time. She has had a spontaneous abortion, a therapeutic abortion, and has two living children born at 39 weeks gestation. G5,T2, P0 ,A2,L2

3. Nadia is pregnant for the sixth time. She has had one spontaneous abortion, one infant born at 32 weeks, two infants born at 39 weeks, one baby born at 41 weeks, and four living children. G6,T3, P1 ,A1 ,L4

4. Jessica is pregnant for the second time. Her first baby was born at 30 weeks gestation and died in the neonatal intensive care nursery. G2,T0,P1 ,A0,L0

5. Susan is pregnant for the first time. She has had no abortions. G1,T0,P0,A0,L0

FILL-IN-THE-BLANK QUESTIONS

What is the importance of each test regarding the care of the pregnant patient?

1. Complete blood count (CBC) to determine overall health & detect anemias
2. Antibody screen to determine wheth
3. Blood typing and Rh identify blood type A, B, AB, O, & Rh status
4. Rubella titer determine whether pt. has immunity
5. Varicella titer _____
6. Hepatitis B determine presence of the antigen to detect in fection
7. HIV and STI screen to detect STDs
8. Papanicolaou (Pap) test cervical cancer
9. Urinalysis to detect bacteria, ketones, glucose, & protein
10. Glucose challenge test screen for gestational diabetes

REVIEW QUESTIONS

1. A 39-year-old patient is 14 weeks gestation. Based on her age and gestation, which diagnostic test/procedure will the health-care provider most likely recommend?
   1. Transvaginal ultrasound
   2. Chorionic villus sampling
   3. Amniocentesis
   4. Pelvis x-ray

   WBC 4500 – 11,000

2. Over-the-counter pregnancy tests are testing the urine for the presence of:
   1. Estrogen
   2. Progesterone
   3. Human chorionic gonadotropin
   4. Luteinizing hormone

3. A patient at 8 weeks gestation has completed the baseline laboratory tests. Which test would indicate that the patient needs to make changes in her diet to have a healthier pregnancy?
   1. WBC count of 8,000
   2. Glucose 99 g/dL
   3. A positive rubella titer
   4. Hemoglobin of 9.2 g/dL

   –3 months, +7 days

4. A patient reports that her last menstrual period began on February 3. Using Naegele's rule, her estimated date of delivery would be:
   1. October 28
   2. November 3
   3. November 10
   4. December 3

5. The student nurse accurately describes quickening with the following statement:
   1. Quickening is when the mother perceives the movement of the fetus.
   2. Quickening is when the fetal heart begins beating.
   3. Quickening is when the embryo attaches to the wall of the uterus.
   4. Quickening is when the labor contractions begin.

6. A 20-year-old patient just found out that her pregnancy test is positive. She confides to the nurse, "This is a terrible time to be pregnant. I am still in college." The best response by the nurse would be:
   1. "Well, everything always seems to work out. Don't worry."
   2. "You have options, such as having an abortion."
   3. "It sounds like you are feeling a little overwhelmed."
   4. "You can always reduce your class load and graduate later."

7. A nurse has taken health histories on four pregnant patients at their first prenatal visit. Which finding should the nurse highlight for the physician or nurse–midwife?
   1. A patient, 8 weeks gestation who had two previous spontaneous abortions
   2. A patient, 10 weeks gestation who is type 1 diabetic
   3. A patient, 10 weeks gestation who has a family history of mental illness
   4. A patient, 8 weeks gestation who smokes

8. The prenatal laboratory tests indicate that a pregnant woman has a negative rubella titer. This indicates that:
   1. She is immune to rubella.
   2. She had the rubella vaccine as a child.
   3. She currently has rubella and is contagious.
   4. She should receive the rubella vaccine after giving birth.

9. A 44-year-old patient states that her home pregnancy test was positive this morning. Which of the following comments by the nurse is appropriate?
   1. "You must be so happy to finally get pregnant!"
   2. "Have you told the baby's father yet?"
   3. "You are a little old to be getting pregnant."
   4. "How do you feel about the results?"

10. When assessing the educational needs for the pregnant patient, appropriate questions would be: (*select all that apply*)
   1. "Have you done any reading about pregnancy?"
   2. "Have any of your friends or family been pregnant lately?"
   3. "What is your marital status?"
   4. "What questions do you have?"
   5. "Did you graduate from high school?"

CONCEPTUAL CORNERSTONE

Even though a pregnancy may be planned and welcomed by a woman and her partner, it is still considered a developmental crisis by human development theorists. Discuss why it is considered a crisis.

PATIENT TEACHING GUIDELINES

Using Internet resources or a laboratory textbook, prepare patient instructions for a glucose challenge test used to screen for gestational diabetes.

POST-CONFERENCE ACTIVITY: CULTURAL CONSIDERATIONS

During post-conference time, share common cultural stereotypes regarding your own ethnic or cultural group. Discuss how stereotyping patients can interfere with providing safe and effective nursing care.

LEARN TO C.U.S. AND THERAPEUTIC COMMUNICATION

Dolores is 23 years old and 32 weeks gestation with her first baby. She arrives at her prenatal appointment 30 minutes late looking messy and disheveled. You note a faint bruise on neck that is covered loosely by a scarf. At previous appointments, she was well groomed and on time. Using the C.U.S. method of communication, discuss your findings with the health-care provider. Using therapeutic communication, plan an appropriate conversation with Dolores.

SAFETY *STAT!*

Sonia is 8 weeks pregnant and is planning to visit her family in Europe. What safety advice can you give Sonia regarding her trip to Europe?

CONCEPT MAP COMPLETION

Complete the concept map with information you have learned about diagnosing pregnancy (Fig. 5.1).

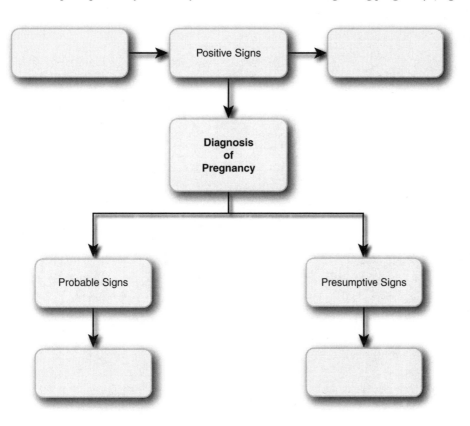

Nursing Care During Pregnancy

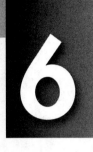

Name: _____

Date: _____

Course: _____

Instructor: _____

REVIEW QUESTIONS

1. A 36 weeks gestation patient calls the obstetrician's office stating, "I think I am making milk, my breasts are leaking." The best response by the nurse is:
   1. "Yes, you are probably making milk; you are close to your due date."
   2. "You should come into the office to be checked for premature labor."
   3. "You are leaking colostrum, which is produced before milk."
   4. "You may have a breast infection; come into the office for an exam."

2. A patient is at 38 weeks gestation. Which discomfort of pregnancy would the nurse expect the patient to exhibit? (*select all that apply*)
   1. Nausea
   2. Backache
   3. Shortness of breath
   4. Ankle edema
   5. Ligament spasm

3. Nausea and vomiting are common during the first trimester. The nurse can provide guidance on managing the discomforts by advising the patient to:
   1. Avoid fruits and fruit drinks.
   2. Eat a large bedtime snack.
   3. Nibble on plain crackers first thing in the morning.
   4. Have a cup of hot decaffeinated coffee before getting out of bed.

4. Toxoplasmosis can be contracted by:
   1. Petting the family cat
   2. Feeding the family cat
   3. Holding the family cat
   4. Cleaning the litterbox for the family cat

5. Forms of exercise appropriate for the pregnant patient are: (*select all that apply*)
   1. Walking
   2. Yoga
   3. Scuba diving
   4. Swimming
   5. Skiing

6. A patient 16 weeks gestation has arrived for her prenatal appointment. What anticipatory guidance would be appropriate for this patient today?
   1. Pain management in labor
   2. Managing leg cramps
   3. Breastfeeding positions
   4. Care of the newborn's umbilical cord

7. A patient is 36 weeks gestation with an uncomplicated pregnancy. She has arrived for her prenatal appointment with her health-care provider. Which of the following tests would be appropriate for her visit today?
   1. Chorionic villi sampling
   2. Culture of vagina and rectum
   3. Contraction stress test
   4. Glucose challenge test

8. The method of transmission of varicella-zoster, also known as *chickenpox*, is:
   1. Airborne
   2. Blood products
   3. Sexual transmission
   4. Raw meat

9. A pregnant patient states that she is experiencing hemorrhoids. An appropriate recommendation by the nurse would be:
   1. Take an over-the-counter laxative.
   2. Increase fiber intake.
   3. Limit fluid intake.
   4. Stop taking the prenatal iron.

10. The nurse is preparing to discuss prenatal nutrition with a pregnant adolescent. The nurse should remember that:
    1. An adolescent is eager to follow all instructions.
    2. An adolescent generally eats well-balanced meals.
    3. An adolescent generally enjoys convenience and fast food.
    4. An adolescent is not concerned with her friends' opinions.

FILL-IN-THE-BLANK QUESTIONS

1. _____Pica_____ is the term for eating non-nutritive foods.

2. HIV is transmitted through ___blood products___, ___body fluids___, and
   _____ _____.

3. _____Nocturia_____ is the term for frequent urination at night.

4. A low level of amniotic fluid is called __Oligohydramnios__.

5. The term __mortality__ refers to deaths.

6. A __nonstress__ __test__ is a test done by applying an external fetal monitor and waiting for the fetus to move.

7. _Polyhydramnios_ is the term for excessive amount of amniotic fluid.

8. Defects of the brain and spinal cord are called _neural_ _tube_ _defects_ .

9. The name for "Husband-Coached Childbirth" is the _Bradley_ method.

10. Couples prepare a _birth_ _plan_ to communicate their desires for their labor and birth experience.

TABLE COMPLETION

Complete the table with information regarding dangerous viruses during pregnancy.

Virus	Method of Transmission	Patient Teaching
Toxoplasmosis	eating raw meat or exposure to cat feces	• Avoid undercooked meat • Avoid cleaning cat litter box • Avoid yardwork that can expose you to cat feces
Cytomegalovirus	• intimate contact with saliva, urine, & other body fluids • sexual contact, breast milk, & placenta	• Use good handwashing after changing diapers or whiping nose • Don't share food, drinks, or eating utensils w/ young children
Herpes Simplex	• STD • can be exposed when passed through the birth canal	• inform healthcare provider of any past outbreaks • practice safe sex
Rubella	• airborne secretions	• know immunization • Avoid exposure to young children in 1st trimester • Obtain vaccine after delivery
Parvovirus B19	• respiratory, blood products, & placenta transmission during pregnancy	• Avoid young children experiencing viral symptoms • handwashing

Continued

Virus	Method of Transmission	Patient Teaching
Varicella-zoster	• airborne	• Avoid any 1 who may have the disease • vaccines for any child once home
Measles	• airborne by caughing & sneezing	• be careful when traveling
HIV	mother → fetus	• HIV testing • take antiretroviral meds as prescribed • Avoid a high-risk lifestyle

CULTURAL CONSIDERATIONS

What suggestions can the nurse make to assist the Asian or Hispanic pregnant patient who practices the hot and cold balance to meet their dietary needs of pregnancy?

make sure they're taking in enough protein
balance protein w/ fruits

PATIENT TEACHING GUIDELINES

Fetal Kick Counts

4x man hour is normal

1. Prepare instructions for teaching a patient how to do a fetal kick count.
2. Using magazines with food pictures, prepare a poster depicting a 24-hour diet intake for a pregnant teenager. Include at least one healthy fast-food meal.

CONCEPTUAL CORNERSTONES

Health Promotion

Using your textbook as a guide, prepare a list of 10 safety tips for pregnant women that will promote a healthy pregnancy and fetus.

1. Good handwashing
2. Avoid undercooked meat
3. Avoid cat feces
4. Avoid smoking/drinks
5. Get flu vaccine
6.
7.
8.
9.
10.

CASE STUDY: LEARN TO C.U.S., THERAPEUTIC COMMUNICATION, AND NURSING PROCESS

Louisa is 34 weeks gestation and arrives in the Emergency Department with symptoms of a urinary tract infection. She mentions that, "The baby is not moving as much today as he was last week." The nurse calls the health-care provider using the C.U.S. method of communication. Plan the conversation:

C: _____

U: _____

S: _____

Answer the following questions regarding the case study.

1. Which diagnostic test would be appropriate in this situation?

   nonstress test

   _____

   _____

2. Using therapeutic communication, how would you discuss your concerns with the patient?

   _____

   _____

   _____

3. Prepare an appropriate nursing diagnosis for this situation with interventions.

   _____

   _____

   _____

CASE STUDY: LABS & DIAGNOSTICS

A patient at 36 weeks gestation has arrived for her prenatal visit. Explain to her the procedure and the importance of the GBS screening.

SAFETY *STAT!*

Prepare a discussion about personal hygiene during pregnancy. Include safety information about tub, shower, hot tub, and sauna use in pregnancy.

CASE STUDY: DRUG FACTS

Jamie is experiencing constipation. She asks the nurse to explain the difference between using a laxative or a stool softener. Which one would be better for her to use? What nonpharmacologic interventions could the nurse suggest?

Nursing Care of the Woman With Complications During Pregnancy

Name: _____

Date: _____

Course: _____

Instructor: _____

POST-CONFERENCE ACTIVITIES

Short Answer Questions

1. Compare and contrast placenta previa and placenta abruption. Discuss signs and symptoms, medical management, and prioritize nursing care for each condition.

   Placenta Previa: placenta planted near opening of cervix
   S/S: painless bright red bleeding, hemorrhaging Intv: bedrest, avoid exercise, sex, C-section if used
   Placenta Abruption: premature seperation of placenta from wall of uterus
   S/S: vaginal bleeding, uterine tenderness, board like abdomen, pain
   Intv: monitor blood loss, document pain level

2. Make a poster comparing and contrasting hyperemesis gravidarum and morning sickness. Provide nonpharmacologic nursing interventions for managing each condition.

   _____

   _____

   _____

   _____

3. Prepare a handout for a newly diagnosed patient with gestational diabetes that explains the process of obtaining a fingerstick blood sugar reading and how to record the information for the health-care provider.

_____

_____

_____

_____

CONCEPTUAL CORNERSTONE
Short Answer Question

Maternal and infant perfusion are important to consider when pregnancy complications occur. When caring for a pregnant patient in the early stages of hypertension, what teaching would you provide to reduce disease advancement?

↓ sodium, ↓ stress

_____

_____

PATIENT TEACHING GUIDELINES
Self-Care after a Spontaneous Abortion
Essay Question

Prepare a teaching plan for a patient following a spontaneous abortion with significant blood loss.

_____

_____

_____

FILL-IN-THE-BLANK QUESTIONS
Abortion

As the instructor lectures over this topic, follow along to fill in the blanks.

1. The term ___abortion___ is used to describe a pregnancy loss prior to the fetus being of viable size and gestational age.

2. A spontaneous ___abortion___ is also known a miscarriage.

3. With a ___threatened___ ___abortion___, the woman experiences abdominal cramping and vaginal bleeding but may not lose the pregnancy.

4. A ___complete___ ___abortion___ occurs when all the uterine contents are expelled.

5. If bleeding does not stop after a spontaneous abortion, a surgical procedure called a ___dilation___ and ___curettage___ may be required.

6. Nursing care includes recognizing the signs of hypovolemic shock due to blood loss. The symptoms that may be exhibited by the patient are ___↓ BP___,
___↑ HR___, ___clammy skin___, ___lightheadedness___, and ___confusion___.

7. The patient should be instructed to report the following warning signs of possible complications following an abortion to her health-care provider: ___heavy, bright red bleeding___, ___foul smelling discharge___, ___fever___, and ___pelvic pain___.

REVIEW QUESTIONS

1. The nurse reviews the chart of a patient scheduled for a contraction stress test. Which condition(s) would be contraindicated for a patient to have a contraction stress test? (*select all that apply*)
   1. Gestational diabetes
   2. Post-term pregnancy of 42 weeks
   3. Third trimester bleeding
   4. Marginal placenta abruption
   5. Oligohydramnios

2. Which patient is at highest risk to develop gestational diabetes?
   1. A 28-year-old African American patient pregnant for the first time who works at a bakery
   2. A 32-year-old Hispanic patient with a BMI of 32.2
   3. A 17-year-old Asian patient who is physically active
   4. A 22-year-old Caucasian patient who works as a teacher

3. The laboratory test used to screen for gestational diabetes is the:
   1. Glucose tolerance test (GTT)
   2. Hemoglobin A1c
   3. Urine glucose test
   4. Random blood sugar test

4. A woman arrives in the emergency department. She states that she is 6 weeks pregnant and is cramping and bleeding vaginally. A speculum exam is done and the examiner notes that the cervix is closed. The probable diagnosis for this woman is:
   1. Threatened abortion
   2. Inevitable abortion
   3. Incomplete abortion
   4. Complete abortion

5. The clinical manifestation of a placenta previa that differs from a placental abruption is:
   1. Bleeding
   2. Uterine contractions
   3. Pain
   4. Cramping

6. Signs of poor perfusion and hypovolemic shock include the following: (*select all that apply*)
   1. Increased blood pressure
   2. Increased pulse
   3. Restlessness
   4. Confusion

7. Select the true statement regarding chronic hypertension and gestational hypertension:
   1. The patient with chronic hypertension never has a blood pressure greater than 140/90 mm Hg.
   2. The patient with gestational hypertension will have her blood pressure return to normal after childbirth.
   3. The patient with chronic hypertension cannot make lifestyle changes to lower her blood pressure.
   4. The patient with gestational hypertension will require blood pressure medications for her entire life.

8. Which short-term goal is appropriate for the patient admitted with hyperemesis gravidarum and the nursing diagnosis of Imbalanced Nutrition: Less than body requirements?
   1. Verbalizes the risk to the fetus
   2. Maintains her present weight
   3. Identifies her favorite foods
   4. Measures her intake hourly

9. The nurse is caring for a patient diagnosed with HELLP syndrome. The nurse knows that the hypertension disorder is characterized by the following: (*select all that apply*)
   1. Elevated liver enzymes
   2. Elevated white blood cells
   3. Low platelet count
   4. Low creatinine levels
   5. Hemolysis of red blood cells

10. Which pregnant patient is most likely to have experienced isoimmunization?
    1. An Rh-positive patient with an Rh-negative partner
    2. An Rh-negative patient with an Rh-negative partner
    3. An Rh-negative patient with no prenatal care and a history of two spontaneous abortions
    4. An Rh-positive patient with no prenatal care and a history of two spontaneous abortions

CROSSWORD PUZZLE

Complications During Pregnancy

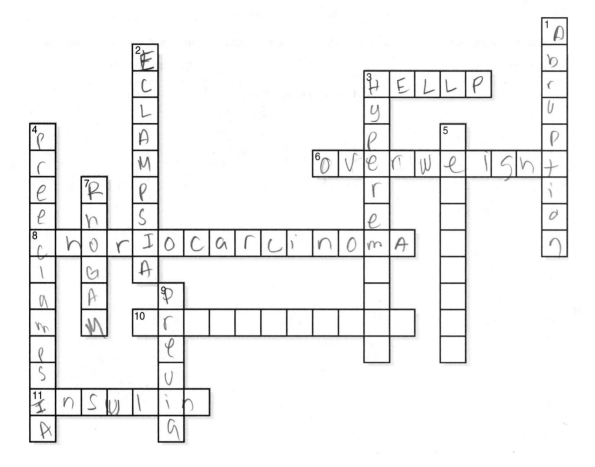

ACROSS

3   hemolysis, elevated liver enzymes, low platelet count
6   a risk factor for gestational diabetes
8   possible complication of a molar pregnancy
10 a sign of preeclampsia
11 a medication used to treat diabetes

DOWN

1   a placenta that detaches too early
2   preeclampsia with the onset of seizures
3   severe vomiting
4   defined as hypertension, proteinuria, and edema
5   the ability for blood to circulate through the body
7   given to women to prevent isoimmunization
9   a low implanted placenta near the cervix

TABLE COMPLETION
Review of Pregnancy-Induced Hypertension (PIH)

Use your textbook and class notes to complete the following table.

Stages of PIH	Medical Signs	Patient Symptoms
Gestational Hypertension	BP of 140/90 or ↑ no proteinuria	
Chronic Hypertension	BP ↑ 140/90 before pregnancy	
Pre-eclampsia	proteinuria, edema BP ↑ 140/90	headaches sudden weight gain
Severe Pre-eclampsia	Abnormal liver function test ↓ urine output proteinuria	blurred vision swollen face, hands, & feet, hyperflexia
Eclampsia	Just like pre-eclampsia, but w/ seizures	
HELLP Syndrome	↑ BP ↑ LDH, AST, ALT, BUN uric acid levels, bilirubin ↓ platelets	

unit THREE

Birth and the Family

8

Process and Stages of Labor and Birth

Name: _____

Date: _____

Course: _____

Instructor: _____

SHORT-ANSWER QUESTION

Note the stages of labor:

Stage 1: _regular uterine contractions → 10cm dilation_

   Phase 1: _latent contractions are 5-20 min apart   dilation to 3cm_

   Phase 2: _active   fetal descent is progressing   dilation to 8_

   Phase 3: _transition   dilation 10_

Stage 2: _pushing, delivery of fetus_

Stage 3: _placenta separation within 30 min_

Stage 4: _uterus is firm, mild uterine cramping_

REVIEW QUESTIONS

1. Which evidence indicates that the patient is experiencing false labor?
   1. The contractions are regular and gradually lasting longer.
   2. The contractions are felt in the back and abdomen.
   3. The contractions go away during a warm shower.
   4. The contractions get stronger when walking.

2. A patient states, "I don't think my water broke, I didn't feel anything. I have noticed a small amount of fluid dripping from my vagina." Which response by the nurse is best?
   1. When the membranes rupture, it is not always a big gush of fluid.
   2. You probably have a uterine infection.
   3. I would not worry about it.
   4. You might be leaking urine.

3. A woman is admitted in labor. Her WBC count is 14,000. The nurse knows that:
   1. The patient has an infection.
   2. The patient has a normal WBC count.
   3. The patient may be anemic.
   4. The patient has not been eating right in pregnancy.

4. A woman was informed by her health-care provider that her baby was in a longitudinal lie. The woman asks the nurse for an explanation. The nurse states:
   1. The baby is lying sideways in your uterus.
   2. The baby is lying at an angle in your uterus.
   3. The baby is lying parallel with your body in the uterus.
   4. The baby is lying face up in your uterus.

5. A patient's mother is assisting her daughter in labor. The mother states, "When I labored, I lay in bed the entire time. Why are you making her walk around and sit in the rocking chair?" The best response by the nurse is:
   1. Your daughter wants to walk around and sit up.
   2. Walking and sitting up have been shown to reduce the length of labor.
   3. It is better for her to sit up.
   4. That was a long time ago; things have changed.

6. Which factors contribute to satisfaction with the birth experience? (*select all that apply*)
   1. Childbirth education classes
   2. Continual one-on-one support during labor
   3. The nurse explaining procedures and progress
   4. The nurse performing all the care for the patient
   5. Previous birth experience of the patient

7. The physician or nurse midwife will become concerned and begin interventions if the placenta does not separate within:
   1. 5 minutes after the birth
   2. 15 minutes after the birth
   3. 30 minutes after the birth
   4. 45 minutes after the birth

8. If the presenting part is the buttocks of the fetus, it is termed a:
   1. Cephalic presentation
   2. Breech presentation
   3. Brow presentation
   4. Transverse presentation

9. A nursing student asks the labor and delivery nurse what the role of the hormone relaxin is during labor. The best response by the nurse is:
   1. "It helps the woman to relax in labor, which shortens labor."
   2. "It causes dilation and effacement to occur before labor begins."
   3. "It causes the fetal heart rate to slow down during hard contractions."
   4. "It softens the cartilage in the pelvis, allowing some stretching to occur."

10. A labor patient asks why she is not hungry even though it has been hours since she last ate. The best response by the nurse is:
   1. During labor, your gastrointestinal system slows down.
   2. During labor, your mind is on the pain, not food.
   3. During labor, you just don't need food.
   4. During labor, you have no room for food in your stomach.

SHORT ANSWER QUESTIONS

1. Neela asks the nurse, "When will I start pushing in labor?"

   in the 2nd stage of labor

   After complete dilation. You will probably feel an urge again

2. Sandra asks the nurse, "How will I know if my water breaks?"

   small trickle or gush, clear w/ no offensive odor

3. Tammi asks the nurse, "How do I time contractions?"

   once you feel a contraction, time how long it is. Time the space
   between your next one

4. Margie asks the nurse, "Does the placenta come out with the baby?"

   No, usually 30 min after birth

5. Sheila asks the nurse, "What causes labor to begin?"

MATCHING EXERCISE

D   1. Acme   A. The part of the fetus that is first to enter the pelvis

E   2. Dilation   B. The "dropping" of the fetus as it descends into the mother's pelvis

J   3. Duration   C. The process of thinning of the cervix

C   4. Effacement   D. The peak of the contraction

G   5. Fetal lie   E. The opening of the closed cervix to ~10 cm

A   6. Fetal presentation   F. Hormone-like substances with a variety of effects on tissues, including the contraction and relaxation of smooth muscle

H   7. Frequency

B   8. Lightening   G. The positioning of the fetus; the most common fetal attitude and the most successful for a vaginal delivery is when the fetus is in a fully flexed position

I   9. Oxytocin

F   10. Prostaglandins

     H. The time between contractions, which is measured from the beginning of one contraction to the beginning of the next contraction

     I. A hormone that is produced in the pituitary gland and secreted into the bloodstream to make the uterus contract

     J. The actual time that a contraction lasts, from beginning to the end

PATIENT TEACHING GUIDELINES
Short Answer Question

1. You are assigned to present a class to a group of women in their third trimester of pregnancy. Prepare an outline of topics that should be addressed.

_____

_____

_____

_____

_____

CASE STUDY
SHORT ANSWER QUESTIONS

Ola is only 1 week from her due date. She arrives at the clinic for a prenatal appointment. She asks the nurse if she might have a bladder infection because she has to urinate frequently.

1. What assessment questions should she ask Ola?

_____

_____

_____

_____

2. What are the possible reasons that Ola is urinating frequently?

_____

_____

_____

_____

3. What could the nurse do to determine whether she is having a urinary tract infection?

_____

_____

_____

_____

POST-CONFERENCE ACTIVITY
Short-Answer Question

List the seven P's of labor and the team members that support the patient in these critical factors of the labor process.

1. _____
2. _____
3. _____
4. _____
5. _____
6. _____
7. _____

LABS & DIAGNOSTICS
Short Answer Question

A patient has just been admitted and objects to having her blood drawn for a CBC. She states, "I have been healthy my entire pregnancy. Why do I need to have blood work done?" What is the best response by the nurse?

_____

_____

_____

_____

THERAPEUTIC COMMUNICATION
Short Answer Question

Cindy is 16 years old and is touring the labor and delivery area. She tells the nurse, "I don't want anyone in the labor room with me. My mom will get on my nerves!"

Using therapeutic communication, what is the best response by the nurse?

_____

_____

_____

_____

Nursing Assessment During Labor

9

Name: _____

Date: _____

Course: _____

Instructor: _____

REVIEW QUESTIONS

1. When caring for a patient in active labor, the patient's vital signs should be assessed every:
   1. 15 minutes
   2. 30 minutes
   3. 1 hour
   4. 2 hours

2. The normal fetal heart rate in labor is:
   1. 100 to 140 bpm
   2. 90 to 160 bpm
   3. 110 to 160 bpm
   4. 110 to 190 bpm

3. Which of the following could cause decreased variability in the fetus during labor? (*select all that apply*)
   1. A sleeping fetus
   2. Fetal hypoxia
   3. An active fetus
   4. A premature fetus
   5. Ruptured membranes

4. When observing the fetal monitor strip, the nurse notes that after the contraction begins, the fetal heart rate drops, with the lowest point occurring after the peak of the contraction. This type of pattern is described as:
   1. An acceleration
   2. An early deceleration
   3. A variable deceleration
   4. A late deceleration

5. The nurse observes the fetal monitor strip and notes that during a contraction, the fetal heart rate drops to the lowest point at the same time the contraction is at a peak. The fetal heart rate then returns to normal by the end of the contraction. The nurse describes this pattern as:
   1. An early deceleration
   2. A variable deceleration
   3. A late deceleration
   4. An episodic deceleration

6. A laboring patient's amniotic membranes have ruptured. The nurse notes that the fluid is greenish in color. The nurse is aware that the green color indicates:
   1. A normal color of amniotic fluid.
   2. The fetus and mother have an Rh incapability problem.
   3. The fetus has experienced possible hypoxia.
   4. The fetus is probably preterm.

7. The nurse has analyzed a fetal monitor strip and determines that the FHR pattern is a Category I pattern. An appropriate action by the nurse would be to:
   1. Document the findings.
   2. Apply oxygen by face mask.
   3. Notify the pediatrician.
   4. Arrange for a Cesarean birth.

8. The patient's husband is very interested in watching the fetal monitor. He has noticed that the heart rate increases when the baby moves. The nurse explains:
   1. "That is nothing for you to worry about."
   2. "That is a positive, expected sign."
   3. "I need to notify the doctor about that problem."
   4. "I'm watching the monitor, don't worry."

9. Management for a variable deceleration may include the following: (*select all that apply*)
   1. Administer oxygen by face mask.
   2. Perform amnioinfusion.
   3. Perform scalp stimulation.
   4. Order a biophysical profile.
   5. Turn the patient to her side.

10. Which of the following laboratory tests may be ordered for the initial assessment and admission of the laboring patient? (*select all that apply*)
    1. CBC
    2. Urinalysis
    3. PT and PTT
    4. Blood type and Rh
    5. Group B strep
    6. Blood cultures
    7. Electrolyte panel

LEARN TO C.U.S

Short Answer Question

A patient has been admitted in early labor. She wants to have a birth experience "free of any invasive procedures and as natural as possible." She has tested positive for group B streptococcus and refuses the intravenous antibiotics ordered by her nurse midwife. Using the C.U.S. method of communication, plan a therapeutic response to the patient.

_____

_____

_____

PATIENT TEACHING GUIDELINES

Short Answer Question

Explain to a newly admitted labor patient the rationale for an intravenous infusion during labor.

an IV is ordered for safety in the event of hemorrhage after birth. It can also be used to administer medication

_____

SAFETY *STAT!*

Short Answer Question

List at least five important safety issues in providing care in labor.

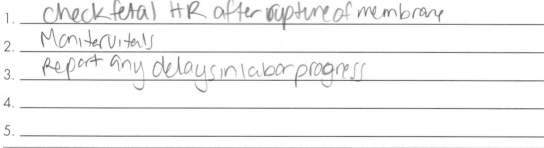

1. Check fetal HR after rupture of membrane
2. Moniter vitals
3. Report any delays in labor progress
4. _____
5. _____

HEALTH PROMOTION

Short Answer Question

Prepare instructions to give a childbirth class on laboring at home during early labor.

_____

_____

_____

CULTURAL CONSIDERATIONS

Short Answer Question

During clinical post conference, share your cultural background and the expectations for support in labor. For example, is the father the major support person or is a sister or mother expected to accompany the patient to the hospital?

Contraction and Deceleration Drawings

1. Early deceleration: Draw a contraction and an early deceleration on the fetal monitor strip (Fig. 9.1).

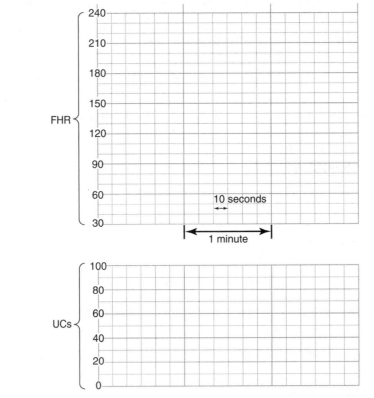

2. Variable deceleration: Draw a contraction and a variable deceleration on the fetal monitor strip (Fig. 9.2).

3. Late deceleration: Draw a contraction and a late deceleration on the fetal monitor strip (Fig. 9.3).

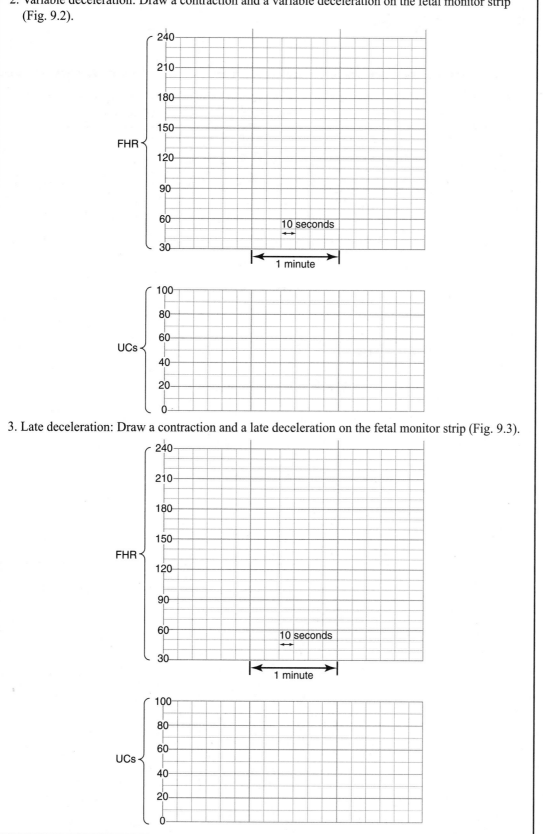

TABLE COMPLETION
Fetal Heart Rate Patterns

Complete the table.

FHR Pattern	Description	Cause	Nursing Interventions
Accelerations	↑ in FHR of 15 beats or above the baseline	normal reassuring change caused by fetus moving	Notify HCP if no accelerations are noted
Early decelerations	gradual decrease in FHR that matches onset of contraction	head compression	none
Variable decelerations	drop in fetal HR that varies w/ timing of contractions	Cord compression that causes hypoxia for fetus	Change pt position, ↑ fluids Administer O₂
Late decelerations	FHR drops after peak of contraction & returns to baseline after contraction	Placental insufficiency, maternal hypotension or uterine hyperactivity	turn pt to side, administer O₂, ↑ fluids

Nursing Care During Labor

10

Name: _____

Date: _____

Course: _____

Instructor: _____

REVIEW QUESTIONS

1. A woman in early labor states, "My sister said she had the urge to push the baby out during her labor. When will I get the urge to push?" The best response by the nurse is:
   1. "I will let you know when it's time to push."
   2. "The urge to push usually comes when the cervix is completely dilated."
   3. "If you have a small baby, you may not get the urge to push at all."
   4. "You can still bear down, even if you don't have the urge to push."

2. You are assigned to a woman in early labor. Appropriate interventions at this time would be: (*select all that apply*)
   1. Allow her to walk.
   2. Provide her with ice chips.
   3. Administer an epidural anesthesia.
   4. Administer butorphanol IV.
   5. Have her sit in a rocking chair.
   6. Provide a lower back massage.

3. A nurse is assessing the newborn to assign a 5 minute Apgar score. The nurse notes that the infant's heart rate is 140 bpm, the respiratory rate is 32 breaths per minute, the baby has good muscle tone with flexion and a good cry, and the baby's feet and hands are slightly blue. The Apgar score assigned for this newborn is:
   1. 7
   2. 8
   3. 9
   4. 10

4. During the first hour after delivery, the patient states, "I am having some uterine cramping." The best responses by the nurse are as follows: (*select all that apply*)
   1. "Do you need medication for the pain?"
   2. "I will call the midwife and report your cramping."
   3. "Everyone cramps a little after childbirth."
   4. "The cramping is caused by the oxytocin in your IV."
   5. "Oh, it will pass in a few minutes."

5. During the first hour after delivery, the patient has soaked two peripads. The nurse:
   1. Is concerned about excessive blood loss and calls the health-care provider.
   2. Knows that this is normal for the first 1 hour and continues to monitor the patient.
   3. Takes another set of vital signs to monitor for signs of shock.
   4. Expects more blood loss and is concerned about a retained placenta.

6. Nursing interventions appropriate for the fourth stage of labor are: (*select all that apply*)
   1. Apply an ice pack to the perineum.
   2. Allow the patient to take a shower.
   3. Assess the fundus.
   4. Assess the amount of vaginal bleeding.
   5. Promote bonding with the newborn.
   6. Administer IM or IV pain medication.

7. During active labor, the patient is restless and changing positions often. The nurse should intervene if the patient is in which position?
   1. Lying on her left side
   2. Sitting on a birthing ball
   3. Standing and leaning on her support person during a contraction
   4. Lying on her back

8. A woman in active labor is using Lamaze breathing techniques with each contraction. The nurse is concerned that she might need additional help with coping with labor because:
   1. She is moaning softly after a contraction.
   2. She has visible tension in her jaw, neck, arms, and hands.
   3. She is asking her support person to massage her back.
   4. She is asking for ice chips between contractions.

9. A thorough pain assessment in labor should include: (*select all that apply*)
   1. Location of the pain
   2. Radiation of the pain
   3. Pattern of the pain
   4. Description of the pain
   5. The support person's perception of the pain
   6. Use of the 1 to 10 pain scale

10. A patient with an epidural anesthesia is 10 cm dilated. Her support person asks why the patient is being allowed to rest and is not pushing. The best response by the nurse is:
    1. "We are letting the epidural wear off a little so that she can push more effectively."
    2. "We will have her start pushing as soon as the doctor arrives."
    3. "Don't worry; I know how to take good care of labor patients."
    4. "My other patient is delivering; she can push when that birth is over."

MATCHING EXERCISE

D   1. Amniotomy

H   2. Analgesia

N   3. Anesthesia

O   4. Apgar score

C   5. Atony

E   6. Doula

M   7. Epidural

L   8. Episiotomy

G   9. Hyperventilation

F   10. Intrathecal space

I   11. Local anesthesia

B   12. Pruritus

J   13. Somatic pain

K   14. Spinal anesthesia

A   15. Visceral pain

A. Pain in internal organs caused by the activation of receptors in the chest, abdomen, or pelvic area that send signals to the spinal cord and on to the brain

B. Intense itching of the skin

C. Lack of normal uterine muscle tone

D. Artificial rupture of the uterine membranes

E. A professional who provides physical, emotional, and informational support to the laboring woman

F. Something that exists within the spinal canal

G. A state that results from an individual's breathing too fast and too deep, which causes a decrease in carbon dioxide in the blood

H. The absence of a normal sense of pain that is achieved by the administration of pain relievers or anesthetics

I. Medication injected to numb an area of the body that is infused by the needle

J. Pain caused by activation of the pain receptors in the body surface or musculoskeletal tissues

K. The placement of a needle into the intrathecal space to inject anesthetic medication

L. An incision into the perineum to enlarge the vaginal opening

M. Anesthesia infused through a catheter between the fourth and fifth vertebrae into the epidural space to decrease pain and perception

N. A drug delivered by gas or injection that causes partial or complete loss of sensation to an area of the body

O. A systematic method of assessing the newborn's heart rate, muscle tone, response to stimuli, and color at 1 minute after birth and again at 5 minutes after birth

TABLE COMPLETION

Provide characteristics of each stage or phase of labor and nursing interventions appropriate for each stage.

Stage or Phase of Labor	Characteristics	Nursing Interventions
Stage 1: Early Phase	Contractions are mild Cervix: 3cm	Implement HCP's orders Assess
Stage 1: Active Phase	Contractions: 2-3min last 60 seconds Cervix: 8cm	• Vitals every 30 min • pain relief • have pt urinate • clear liquids
Stage 1: Transition	Contractions: 2-3 min lasts 60-90 seconds Cervix: 10cm	• Stay w/ pt. • Assess
Stage 2: Pushing and Birth	• pt has urge to push • fetus is delivered	• Catch pt. • prepare room for delivery
Stage 3: Birth through Placenta Delivery	• mild cramping as placenta is delivered	

SHORT ANSWER QUESTIONS

1. How can the nurse provide support to the patient's labor partner?

   _____

   _____

   _____

2. How can the nurse establish a therapeutic relationship with a newly admitted labor patient?

   _____

   _____

   _____

LEARN TO C.U.S.

Short Answer Question

Lori is in labor with her fourth child and is 8 cm dilated. According to her birth plan, she has wanted a medication-free labor and delivery but the contractions have become very intense. She is now asking for IV pain medication. The nurse knows that Lori's labor could progress to delivery very quickly because she is delivering her fourth baby. The nurse uses the C.U.S. method to communicate with Lori and her husband.

C: _____

U: _____

S: _____

THERAPEUTIC COMMUNICATION

Short Answer Questions

Using therapeutic communication, re-write the nontherapeutic nurse response.
  Patient: "I don't want my mother in here while I am in labor."
  Nurse: "Why?"

  Nurse: _____
  Patient: "She fusses over me like I am a child. I have a birth plan."
  Nurse: "I am sure she just wants to help."

  Nurse: _____
  Patient: "I want an epidural. She had me without medication and thinks I should do the same thing."
  Nurse: "Your mother may know what's best for you."

  Nurse: _____

CULTURAL CONSIDERATIONS

Short Answer Question

How can the nurse incorporate a couple's cultural practices into labor care?

_____

_____

_____

HEALTH PROMOTION

Short Answer Question

Develop a teaching plan for pregnant teenagers about nonpharmacological comfort measures in labor. Include a list of items they may want to bring from home.

_____

_____

_____

SAFETY *STAT!*: CASE STUDY

Short Answer Question.

The following paragraph has many safety issues. List each safety issue and explain why it is a safety concern for this patient.

Yvonne is in labor with her first baby. She is quietly resting in bed on her back. On the bedside table are a cola and a tuna fish sandwich she brought from home in case she became hungry in labor. Her contractions are every 3 minutes and last 60 seconds. A few minutes ago, her water broke and she plans to tell the nurse the next time she comes in the room. Yvonne wants a medication-free labor but brought a few aspirin with her "just in case." Yvonne's husband just stepped out of the room to make a phone call. When he returns, she wants him to help her to the bathroom because she is feeling pressure and might need to have a bowel movement.

1. _____

2. _____

3. _____

4. _____

5. _____

PATIENT TEACHING GUIDELINES: CASE STUDY

Essay Question

Cindy is in early labor and has a few questions for the nurse about epidurals. Cindy asks, "Can I move around after I get an epidural? How good is the pain relief? I heard I might get itchy with an epidural. Is that true? Is it safe for the baby?"

How should the nurse answer Cindy's questions?

_____

_____

_____

_____

_____

Nursing Care of the Woman With Complications During Labor and Birth

11

Name: _____

Date: _____

Course: _____

Instructor: _____

REVIEW QUESTIONS

1. After the delivery of a 7 pound male, the placenta fails to deliver within 30 minutes. The nurse midwife looks up at the nurse and states, "We have a placenta accreta." The nurse expects the patient to:
   1. Develop hypertension
   2. Begin seizure activity
   3. Begin hemorrhaging
   4. Experience hyperthermia

2. Which of the following is considered a vaginal delivery emergency?
   1. A primigravida patient has been pushing for more than 1 hour.
   2. The head is born but the shoulders cannot pass under the pubic arch.
   3. The head is in the occiput posterior position.
   4. The placenta delivers 20 minutes after the baby.

3. A primigravida is admitted to the labor and delivery unit. Her membranes have ruptured, she is 1 cm dilated, is 20% effaced, and is not having contractions. She asks the nurse, "Do I get the epidural now? I really don't want any pain." The *best* responses by the nurse are: (*select all that apply*)
   1. "You might as well accept that you will have pain with labor and delivery."
   2. "We can't give the epidural until you are well established in labor or it may slow your labor."
   3. "I will call the anesthesiologist immediately and get started on it."
   4. "I can help you cope with the pain until the epidural is started."
   5. "What can I do to help you relax?"

4. A patient is experiencing severe back pain due to a posterior presentation of the fetus. Which of the following nursing interventions will be effective in this situation? (*select all that apply*)
   1. Place the patient in Trendelenburg's position.
   2. Place the patient on her left side.
   3. Place the patient on her right side.
   4. Place the patient supine.
   5. Encourage the patient to stand while leaning forward.

5. A patient suddenly begins having difficulty breathing, becomes confused, and is hypotensive. The nurse suspects:
   1. Amniotic fluid embolism
   2. Placenta abruption
   3. Placenta accreta
   4. Uterine prolapse

6. During a vaginal delivery, the physician states that a shoulder dystocia is occurring. Which intervention may be expected of the nurse?
   1. Place the patient in Trendelenburg's position.
   2. Call the laboratory for an immediate blood type and crossmatch.
   3. Prepare the vacuum extractor for the health-care provider to use.
   4. Assist the woman to flex her thighs upon her abdomen.

7. A patient has been admitted to the labor and delivery department. No fetal heart tones can be located. She states that she has not felt the baby move for 1 day. The ultrasound reveals that the fetus has died. The patient says, "Can you repeat the tests again, just to be sure?" The patient is exhibiting which stage of grieving?
   1. Anger
   2. Acceptance
   3. Denial
   4. Guilt

8. Risk factors associated with macrosomia include: (*select all that apply*)
   1. Maternal obesity
   2. Gestational diabetes
   3. Asian descent
   4. Hispanic decent
   5. Postmaturity
   6. Polyhydramnios

9. A patient is receiving magnesium sulfate for preterm labor. Which sign or symptom noticed by the nurse would cause the nurse to stop the infusion?
   1. DTRs 1+
   2. Respiratory rate of 10
   3. Blood pressure of 108/60 mm Hg
   4. The patient is drowsy

10. Risk factors for a prolapsed cord include: (*select all that apply*)
    1. Fetal head at 1+ station when the membranes rupture
    2. Multiple gestation
    3. Postmaturity
    4. Prematurity
    5. Breech

11. A priority intervention following a precipitous delivery of a newborn would be:
    1. Call the doctor or nurse midwife.
    2. Reassure the patient.
    3. Prevent hypothermia of the infant.
    4. Apply ID band to the infant.

12. A patient is receiving indomethacin. The nurse is aware that a common side effect of this
    medication is:
    1. Decreased respirations
    2. Gastrointestinal upset
    3. Rash
    4. Tachycardia

THERAPEUTIC COMMUNICATION

Short Answer Questions

Write a therapeutic response to the following patient comments.

1. "I can't believe this is happening to me. My baby is dead?"

_____

_____

2. "I can't be on bed rest at home. I have a 2-year-old."

_____

_____

3. "I must have caused this preterm labor when I ate those hot peppers."

_____

_____

4. "My grandmother says that a baby born at 7 months has a better chance than a baby born
   at 8 months."

_____

_____

5. "My doctor said the baby is getting big, and I don't have a large pelvis. Shouldn't we just get going
   with the Cesarean?"

_____

_____

ILLUSTRATION EXERCISE

Identify the type of placenta problem.

1. Figure 11.1: _Placental abruption_____

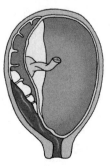

2. Figure 11.2: _placenta previa_

Internal os
Blood
External os

🔴 DRUG FACTS

Short Answer Questions

Patients on the labor and delivery unit are to receive the following medications. Explain to the patients, in easy to understand language, the reason for each medication.

1. Magnesium sulfate

   relaxes smooth muscle & decreases uterine activity slowing or stopping contraction

2. Indomethacin

   prostaglandin inhibitor, stops production of cytokines that cause labor to begin

3. Betamethasone

   prevents neonatal respiratory distress

4. Nifidipine

   inhibits smooth muscle contractions of the uterus

5. Progesterone

   relaxes uterine muscles & prevents contractions

ILLUSTRATION EXERCISE

Identify the type of presentation.

1. Figure 11.3: _____

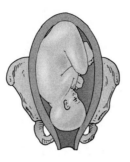

2. Figure 11.4: _____ breech _____

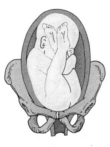

3. Figure 11.5: _____

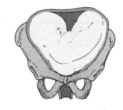

FILL-IN-THE-BLANK QUESTIONS

1. A patient has a history of spontaneous miscarriages in the second trimester. The nurse suspects that the patient may have _incompetent cervix_. The common management of this condition is _cervical cerclage_.

2. A patient experiences a rupture of her membranes. The nurse notes that only a small amount of fluid was expelled and the patient is 39 weeks gestation but her uterus is smaller than her dates indicate. The nurse suspects _oligohydramnios_ and is aware that the fetus may be _small for gestational age_.

3. A nurse is performing a vaginal cervical examination on a newly admitted laboring patient. The nurse notes on the exam that the cervix is 4 cm dilated and 75% effaced. The membranes are intact, and the nurse felt a foot move inside the intact membranes during the examination. The nurse reports the fetal position as _footling breech_. The nurse is aware that the patient is at high risk of _umbilical cord prolapse_ if the membranes rupture. The nurse is aware that a _C-section_ birth is likely for this patient.

4. The _____pelvis_____ may contribute to dysfunctional labor because the pelvic bones may be too narrow.

5. A woman may experience hypotonic labor contractions (_____power_____) that are not effective to produce cervical dilation.

6. The woman's _____psyche_____ contributes to labor progression and her management of anxiety.

7. The fetal _____presentation_____ of brow, breech, or shoulder can slow labor progression.

8. A patient is experiencing a leakage of clear fluid, vaginal discharge, and pelvic pressure but no contractions. To verify that the fluid is amniotic fluid, the nitrazine paper turns purple, confirming the diagnosis. The nurse knows that the patient has _____premature rupture of membranes_____ and the most serious complication for this condition is _____infection_____.

9. Amniotic fluid volume is an indication of fetal well-being. An abnormally high level of fluid is termed _____polyhydramnios_____ and an abnormally low level of amniotic fluid is termed _____oligohydramnios_____.

10. A patient is admitted in early labor. She is scheduled for a repeat Cesarean birth tomorrow. She is a gravida 5, para 4, and her youngest child is 14 months old. Based on this information, the nurse is aware that the patient is a risk for _____uterine rupture_____.

11. Coagulation tests that may be ordered by the physician while caring for a patient with a suspected amniotic fluid embolus are: _____PT, PTT, fibrinogen, D-dimer_____

LEARN TO C.U.S.

Short Answer Question

The labor and delivery nurse has just admitted a patient to the unit. The patient's history indicates that she is a primigravida, obese, diabetic, and her due date was 2 weeks ago. She began having contractions at home 8 hours ago. The patient is having strong contractions every 3 minutes lasting 60 seconds. Her membranes ruptured at home 2 hours ago and the fluid was clear. The nurse notes on vaginal examination that the patient is 5 cm dilated and the fetal head is at −1 station. The nurse is concerned about possible fetal macrosomia based on the patient's history and the assessment information that the fetus is not engaged in the pelvis despite strong contractions and ruptured membranes. The nurse uses the C.U.S. method to communicate with the nurse midwife.

C: _____

U: _____

S: _____

MATCHING EXERCISE

_I_ 1. The uterus inverts and prolapses through the vaginal opening after delivery.

_B._ 2. The use of sutures around the cervix to prevent it from opening.

_C_ 3. Infection of the amniotic and chorionic membranes.

_A_ 4. Artificial rupture of the amniotic sac.

_D_ 5. The death of a fetus.

_J._ 6. The nonsurgical opening of the uterus.

_E_ 7. Benign uterine tumors.

_H_ 8. A situation in which the fetal shoulders get wedged in the pelvis after the head is delivered.

_F_ 9. A newborn with a birth weight greater than 4000 to 4500 g

_G_ 10. The umbilical cord around the neck of the fetus

A. Amniotomy

B. Cerclage

C. Chorioamnionitis

D. Fetal demise

E. Fibromyomas

F. Macrosomia

G. Nuchal cord

H. Shoulder dystocia

I. Uterine inversion

J. Uterine rupture

POST-CONFERENCE QUESTIONS AND ACTIVITIES

Short Answer Questions

1. A patient's husband runs up to a group of student nurses as they leave the hospital at the end of their clinical day. He shouts, "My wife is having a baby right now in our car! Please help me!" What should the student nurses do to provide for safety of the patient and her baby?

   _____

   _____

2. How can the nurse meet the psychosocial needs of the patient in preterm labor?

   _____

   _____

3. A patient has been admitted to the labor and delivery department for labor induction. She is 42 weeks gestation. She states that she is unsure of whether she wants to have her labor induced. As the nurse, how would you explain the risks of postmaturity for the fetus?

_____

_____

4. A patient is in active labor. She is dilated 4 cm and complains of severe low back pain during each contraction. The nurse suspects that the fetus is in the posterior position and suggests the following interventions:

_____

_____

5. A patient has just been admitted to labor and delivery. She is having contractions every 3 minutes with duration of 60 seconds. She is bleeding vaginally and complaining of severe abdominal pain. The nurse suspects that the patient may have a placental abruption and appropriate nursing interventions would be:

_____

_____

TABLE COMPLETION
Labor-Related Complications

Complication	Signs	Nursing Care
Dysfunctional Labor (failure to progress or cephalopelvic disproportion)	Slow dilation despite contractions, Slow descent of fetus	• pt. position changes • empty bladder • provide non pharmacological comfort measures
Breech	feet or buttocks palpated during vaginal exam	• examine for prolapsed cord • report findings to HCP
Umbilical Cord Prolapse	Sudden onset of variable decelerations or bradycardia	• position pt in Trendlenburg • Administer O2 • C-section
Uterine Rupture	• complaint of uterine pain • fetal bradycardia	• C-section • notify HCP • administer O2

CONCEPT MAP COMPLETION

CONCEPTUAL CORNERSTONE: ANXIETY IN PREGNANCY

A normal uncomplicated pregnancy can cause some level of anxiety for any woman. However, a woman with a complication of pregnancy, such as preterm labor, can experience extreme anxiety over the outcome of the pregnancy and the health of her baby. Complete the concept map with nonpharmacological nursing interventions to reduce anxiety (Fig. 11.6).

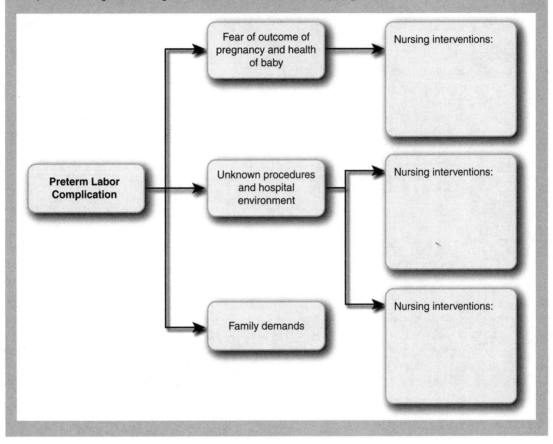

Birth-Related Procedures

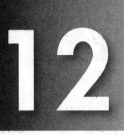

Name: _____

Date: _____

Course: _____

Instructor: _____

REVIEW QUESTIONS

1. Following a forceps delivery, the nurse will be monitoring for which possible maternal complication?
   1. Uterine atony
   2. Placenta accreta
   3. Bleeding from a vaginal tear
   4. Maternal exhaustion

2. The nurse is aware that oxytocin is safe for labor induction because:
   1. Only qualified nurses can administer the medication.
   2. It has a very short half-life and clears the system quickly.
   3. Only small doses of the medication are infused.
   4. The dosage is double-checked by a pharmacist.

3. Potential complications of an external cephalic version include: (*select all that apply*)
   1. Twisting of the umbilical cord
   2. Placenta accreta
   3. Placenta abruptio
   4. Brachial plexus injury
   5. Rupture of amniotic membranes

4. Indications for labor induction include: (*select all that apply*)
   1. Post-term pregnancy
   2. Fetal demise
   3. Prolonged rupture of membranes
   4. Twin pregnancy
   5. Convenience for the patient

5. A patient is being prepared for a Cesarean birth after a long labor. She states, "I am very nervous about surgery. When I had knee surgery, the nurse gave me medication in my IV to relax me. When do I get that medication?" The best response by the nurse is:
   1. "There's no time for that!"
   2. "It wouldn't be safe for the baby."
   3. "I don't have a doctor's order for any medication."
   4. "Don't worry, you won't feel a thing."

6. The nurse knows that it is important that the patient have an empty bladder when undergoing a vacuum extraction assisted birth because:
   1. The bladder might get cut by the vacuum extractor devise.
   2. The patient may be uncomfortable because she needs to urinate.
   3. An empty bladder allows more room in the pelvis.
   4. Urine leaking during the procedure can cause contamination of the perineum.

7. Assign a Bishop score from the following information: cervix is dilated 1 cm, 30% effaced, and of medium consistency in a posterior position, and the fetal head is at –1 station.
   1. 3 points
   2. 4 points
   3. 5 points
   4. 6 points

8. Contraindications to cervical ripening include: (*select all that apply*)
   1. Breech presentation
   2. 40 weeks gestation
   3. Placenta previa
   4. Active herpes infection
   5. Bishop score of 5 points

9. After an amniotomy, the nurse assesses the fetal heart rate (FHR) because:
   1. The fetus may have changed position.
   2. The contractions become stronger.
   3. The umbilical cord can prolapse or become compressed.
   4. The FHR may be more difficult to hear.

10. Nursing care for a patient undergoing labor induction with oxytocin includes: (*select all that apply*)
    1. Inserting a Foley catheter for urinary drainage.
    2. Preparing the infusion connected "piggy back" through a pump.
    3. Monitoring for tachysytole.
    4. Stopping the infusion if a non-reassuring FHR is noted.
    5. Positioning the patient in lateral recumbent position for 30 minutes.

TRUE OR FALSE QUESTIONS

1. __F__ An amniotomy is used to determine if the cervix is favorable for induction of labor.

2. __T__ Augmentation of labor is the stimulation of hypotonic uterine contractions.

3. __T__ An active herpes infection is a contraindication for cervical ripening.

4. __F__ Prostaglandin gel is applied to the uterine fundus to induce labor.

5. __F__ Tachysytole poses no risk to the fetus.

6. __T__ A vacuum extraction devise can cause a cephalohematoma on the fetal head.

7. __F__ An epidural is effective for pain management during a Cesarean birth.

8. __F__ A woman who has had three Cesarean births is a good candidate for a vaginal birth after previous Cesarean (VBAC).

9. _T_ Maternal obesity is a risk factor for a Cesarean birth.

10. _T_ A laceration of the vagina is a possible complication from a forceps delivery.

FILL-IN-THE-BLANK QUESTIONS

1. The Bishop score indicates if the __cervix__ is ready to respond to efforts to stimulate labor.

2. A __Foley's__ __Catheter__ _____ is a mechanical method of ripening the cervix and stimulating labor.

SHORT ANSWER QUESTIONS

1. The purpose of an external cephalic version is to _place the fetus in a head down presentation_.

2. Amnioinfusion is _the process of infusing fluid into the uterine cavity to treat cord compression_.

3. Possible complications of amnioinfusion include:

   • _____

   • _____

   • _____

   • _____

   • _____

   • _____

   • _____

CASE STUDY

SHORT ANSWER QUESTIONS

Tera has been in labor for several hours. She is 4 cm dilated. Her labor is progressing slowly because her contractions are hypotonic and irregular. The obstetrician has performed an amniotomy.

1. What is the appropriate nursing care following an amniotomy?

   _____

   _____

   _____

2. What patient teaching would be appropriate?

   _____

   _____

   _____

POST-CONFERENCE ACTIVITIES

CONCEPTUAL CORNERSTONE: COLLABORATION AND TEAM WORK

Short Answer Questions

1. List examples of interprofessional collaboration that you have encountered in the health-care setting.

_____

_____

_____

2. List examples of nurse-to-nurse collaboration that you have observed in the health-care setting.

_____

_____

_____

3. List examples of nurse-to-patient collaboration that you have observed in the health-care setting.

_____

_____

_____

PATIENT TEACHING GUIDELINES: CESAREAN BIRTH

Short Answer Questions

A patient has been laboring for hours with little progress on cervical dilation. She has agreed to a Cesarean delivery. List the main teaching points to quickly prepare her for the Cesarean birth.

_____

_____

_____

CONCEPTUAL CORNERSTONE: STRESS

Short Answer Question

The team is working quickly to prepare a patient for an emergency Cesarean delivery. List nursing interventions to reduce stress for the patient in order to promote a safe delivery of the fetus.

_____

_____

_____

THERAPEUTIC COMMUNICATION

Short Answer Questions

Prepare a therapeutic answer for the patient in the following scenario:

Thea is 25 years old and 41 weeks gestation with her first baby. She is admitted to the labor and delivery area for labor induction with oxytocin.

Thea: "I really don't get it. What's wrong with being overdue anyway? I prefer a natural approach."

Nurse: _____

_____

Thea: "I've heard that oxytocin is very painful."

Nurse: _____

_____

Thea: "I've read that inductions don't always work. Do you think I will end up having a C-section?"

Nurse: _____

_____

Thea: "What if I can't handle the pain?"

Nurse: _____

_____

LEARN TO C.U.S.

Short Answer Question

The labor and delivery nurse is caring for a patient receiving an induction of labor with oxytocin. After the oxytocin begins infusing, the patient has two contractions that last 110 seconds and the FHR decelerated after the peak of each contraction. The FHR returned to normal after the contraction. The nurse is concerned and uses the C.U.S. method to communicate with the health-care provider.

C: _____

U: _____

S: _____

TEAM WORKS

Short Answer Question

Preparing a patient for an emergency Cesarean requires the collaboration of the entire team in order to ensure a safe birth for the mother and fetus. List all the possible members of team.

1. _____

2. _____

3. _____

4. _____

5. _____

6. _____

CASE STUDY
SHORT ANSWER QUESTION

Sofia, gravida 1, was just admitted to the labor and delivery department for induction of labor. Her due date was 3 days ago. The nurse performs a cervical exam and finds that Sofia's cervix is closed, 20% effaced, of medium consistency, and located in the mid-position. The fetus is at a −2 station. What

is Sofia's Bishop Score? Is an induction of labor likely to be successful? _____

_____

_____

_____

_____

unit FOUR

Postpartum Period and the Family

Physiological and Behavioral Adaptations During the Postpartum Period

13

Name: _____

Date: _____

Course: _____

Instructor: _____

REVIEW QUESTIONS

1. A woman who does not want to breastfeed has been counseled about how to decrease milk production. Which of the following actions demonstrates that the teaching was effective?
   1. The woman puts on a tight-fitting bra.
   2. The woman stands in the shower for a long time with warm water running over her breasts.
   3. The woman expresses a small amount of milk from her breast with her hand.
   4. The woman massages her breasts every hour.

2. The nurse notes that a patient is bleeding heavily 2 hours after delivery. Abdominal palpation reveals that the uterus is leaning to the right of the abdominal midline and the bladder is palpable. The first action the nurse should take is:
   1. Call the health-care provider.
   2. Change the patient's peripads.
   3. Ask the patient to urinate and empty her bladder.
   4. Massage the uterus.

3. The nurse is reviewing the patient medical record and calls the health-care provider regarding which blood value?
   1. WBC: 18,000 cells/mm^3
   2. RBC: 4,500,000 cells/mm^3
   3. Hemoglobin: 9.0 g/dL
   4. Platelets: 250,000 per mm^3

4. A postpartum patient asks when she will stop having the vaginal discharge. The best response by the nurse is:
   1. 1 to 2 weeks
   2. 1 to 3 weeks
   3. 1 to 5 weeks
   4. 1 to 6 weeks

5. A nurse is planning care for a patient in the "taking-hold" phase of maternal role attainment. The nurse should include which of the following in the plan of care?
   1. Assist the patient with her shower.
   2. Provide her with nutritious snacks.
   3. Provide her with positive encouragement.
   4. Allow her to take a long nap.

6. A patient's husband calls the postpartum unit the day after the patient went home. He states, "I don't understand. I just made a comment about her still being in her robe and she burst into tears. Is there something wrong with her?" The best response by the nurse is:
   1. "You need to be more kind in your comments."
   2. "That's normal; it's called the postpartum blues."
   3. "Just leave her alone, she'll get over it."
   4. "She must have been really upset with you."

7. Twenty minutes after delivery, the patient begins to shake uncontrollably. The best response by the nurse is to:
   1. Increase the rate of IV fluids.
   2. Ask the patient if she is having a seizure.
   3. Provide a warm blanket and reassurance.
   4. Call the health-care provider.

8. A postpartum patient is being discharged. She states to the nurse, "My 3-year-old is so excited for me to bring home her new baby sister." An appropriate response by the nurse would be:
   1. "That won't last long."
   2. "It's nice to see children excited about a new baby in the family."
   3. "You will have a little helper. She may want to play mother to the new baby."
   4. "She may be excited, but do expect a little jealousy and adjustment to occur."

9. Upon examination of a 1 day postpartum patient, the nurse expects to see: (*select all that apply*)
   1. The fundus one finger-breadth below the umbilicus
   2. Warm, engorged breasts
   3. The new mother doing all the newborn care
   4. Rubra lochia
   5. An episode of the postpartum blues exhibited by the patient's tears

10. A new father is observed to be staring at his new son. This behavior is termed:
    1. Bonding
    2. Engagement
    3. Engrossment
    4. Attachment

FILL-IN-THE BLANK QUESTIONS

1. The lochia ___serosa___ is pink or brown in color and may last for 4 to 9 days.

2. ___Exfoliatia___ is the sloughing of dead tissue at the placental site, leaving the site without scar tissue.

3. The folds of the vaginal tissue are called ___rugae___.

4. After delivery, the hormone ___relaxin___ begins to subside, which causes some hip and joint discomfort.

5. The process of the uterus returning to its normal size is called ___involution___.

6. ___Kegel___ exercises can help the perineum to tighten and regain tone.

7. The last phase of maternal role attainment is called ___Letting go___.

8. Cramping after delivery is called ___after___ ___pains___.

9. The postpartum woman's body begins to remove excessive fluid by ___diuresis___ and by ___diaphoresis___.

10. The ___postpartum___ ___blues___ is a normal temporary psychological condition that many women experience.

POST-CONFERENCE ACTIVITY: CULTURAL CONSIDERATIONS

During clinical at the postpartum unit, briefly interview a patient about her cultural beliefs about bonding and postpartum care. Share your findings at post-conference time.

THERAPEUTIC COMMUNICATION

Short Answer Question

A new mother is expressing anxiety regarding her ability to care for her infant. The nurse has an important role in providing encouragement. List three phrases the nurse could say to the new mother to encourage her and relieve her anxiety.

1. _____

2. _____

3. _____

MATCHING EXERCISE

_J_ 1. Pink or brown uterine discharge that lasts for 4 to 9 days.

_F_ 2. An attitude of total focus often seen in new fathers.

_E_ 3. The passage of large amounts of urine.

_H_ 4. The final stage of uterine sloughing, a yellow white discharge.

_B_ 5. The emotional and physical attachment between a mother and her newborn.

_I_ 6. Bright red uterine discharge that lasts 1 to 3 days.

_A_ 7. The incorporation of the new baby into the family unit.

_G_ 8. The large upper part of the uterus.

_C_ 9. The first fluid produced by the breasts after childbirth.

_D_ 10. Separation of the abdominal muscles.

A. Attachment
B. Bonding
C. Colostrum
D. Diastasis recti
E. Diuresis
F. Engrossment
G. Fundus
H. Lochia alba
I. Lochia rubra
J. Lochia serosa

SAFETY *STAT!*

Short Answer Question

A postpartum patient has increased levels of fibrinogen. This can predispose the patient to blood clots. List nursing interventions that prevent the formation of blood clots.

1. _____

2. _____

3. _____

TRUE OR FALSE QUESTIONS

1. __F__ Family dynamics do not change when a new baby is born into a family.

2. __T__ Immediately after birth, estrogen and progesterone levels begin to drop.

3. __F__ After the placenta is delivered, the fundus cannot be palpated.

4. __T__ By day 14 postpartum, the cervix is closed.

5. __T__ Kegel exercises can help to restore tone to the perineal area.

6. __T__ The first menstrual period for a postpartum woman can occur anytime from 6 to 12 weeks after delivery.

7. __F__ Women who do not choose to breastfeed can apply warm packs to the breasts to reduce pain.

8. __T__ Women can develop hemorrhoids during late pregnancy and while pushing to deliver the baby.

9. __F__ Expected blood loss following a vaginal delivery is 1000 mL.

10. __T__ A full bladder can interfere with involution of the uterus.

11. __T__ In the "taking-in" phase, a new mother may be very centered on her own needs.

12. __F__ The "taking-in" phase is a good time to begin teaching about newborn care.

13. __T__ Most women experience the postpartum blues for a day or two.

14. __T__ The father should be encouraged to provide newborn care in the hospital.

15. __F__ Well-prepared siblings will not exhibit signs of jealousy over the new sibling.

HEALTH PROMOTION: RETURNING GASTROINTESTINAL FUNCTION

Short Answer Question

During pregnancy, many women experience constipation and, after delivery, it may take a while for gastrointestinal function to return to normal. List appropriate nursing interventions to promote gastrointestinal health.

1. _____

2. _____

3. _____

4. _____

5. _____

TABLE COMPLETION
Drug Facts: Postpartum Medications

Two commonly prescribed medications on the postpartum unit are anti-inflammatories and stool softeners. Complete the table with information that you would give the patient when you administer these medications.

Medication	Purpose	Possible Side Effects
Ibuprofen	↓ inflammation & control pain	GI upset
Docusate	Softens stool & ↓ pain from 1st bowel movement	Abdominal cramps & diarrhea

Assessment and Care of the Family After Birth

Name: _____

Date: _____

Course: _____

Instructor: _____

REVIEW QUESTIONS

1. The labor and delivery nurse is completing an assessment of a patient 1 hour after delivery and prior to transfer to the postpartum unit. The vital signs are as follows: B/P: 122/70, P: 80, R: 18, Temperature: 98.4°F (36.9°C). The fundus is firm and is located in the midline halfway between the symphysis pubis and the umbilicus. The nurse notes heavy rubra lochia with a few pea-sized clots on the peripad. At the episiotomy site, edema is noted. The nurse should: (*select all that apply*)
   1. Document the findings.
   2. Notify the health-care provider of the abnormal findings.
   3. Offer an ice pack for the episiotomy site.
   4. Assist the patient to the bathroom to urinate.
   5. Allow the patient to be transferred to the postpartum unit.
   6. Change the peripad before transfer to the postpartum unit.

2. The nurse should intervene if the student nurse is observed to be:
   1. Assisting a patient to the bathroom 6 hours after delivery.
   2. Massaging the fundus with one hand and pulling the peripad down with the other hand.
   3. Assisting the patient with breastfeeding and latch-on 30 minutes after delivery.
   4. Teaching a patient how apply a peripad from the front to the back.

3. Which of the following *T*s are possible causes of postpartum hemorrhage? (*select all that apply*)
   1. Time
   2. Tone
   3. Tissue
   4. Technique
   5. Thrombin
   6. Trauma

4. A patient confides to the nurse that she is feeling "strange" and that she hears voices telling her that "my baby is in danger from the devil." The nurse should: (*select all that apply*)
   1. Ask her if she feels like hurting herself or her baby.
   2. Staying with the woman and her baby until relieved by another nurse or health-care provider.
   3. Notifying the health-care provider immediately.
   4. Reassuring the woman that those thoughts will disappear in a few days.
   5. Inform her partner that she needs to be "watched for a few days."

5. Nursing interventions for a patient with a urinary tract infection include: (*select all that apply*)
   1. Encouraging the patient to increase fluid intake.
   2. Encouraging the patient to increase fiber in the diet.
   3. Teaching the patient to apply a peripad from front to back.
   4. Administering antibiotics as ordered.
   5. Instructing the patient to avoid carbonated drinks.

6. Risk factors for thrombophlebitis include: (*select all that apply*)
   1. Premature rupture of membranes
   2. Obesity
   3. History of varicose veins
   4. Hypertension
   5. Smoking
   6. Prolonged bed rest

7. Nursing care to prevent thrombus formation includes: (*select all that apply*)
   1. Maintaining bed rest
   2. Ambulation as soon as possible
   3. Applying compression stockings or sequential devices
   4. Elevating the legs whenever possible
   5. Decreasing fluid intake

8. The laboratory test that is ordered to monitor the effectiveness of anticoagulant therapy is:
   1. CBC
   2. INR
   3. HCT
   4. HCG

9. Signs of postpartum depression include:
   1. Breastfeeding problems
   2. Fatigue
   3. Anhedonia
   4. Hallucinations

10. A 15-year-old patient gave birth 2 hours ago. She is planning to raise the baby with the help of her parents. At this time, she states that she is exhausted and is refusing to hold the baby. She asks the nurse to return the baby to the nursery. The nurse should:
    1. Insist that she keep the baby in her room because it would be good for bonding.
    2. Show her how to diaper and wrap up the baby for warmth.
    3. Allow her to rest and take the baby to the nursery.
    4. Inform her that all the mothers keep their babies in the room.

SHORT ANSWER QUESTION

The mnemonic BUBBLE LE is used to remember the steps of the postpartum assessment. Fill in the word for each letter.

B _____

U _____

B _____

B _____

L _____

E _____

L _____

E _____

MATCHING EXERCISE

_____ 1. Anhedonia

_____ 2. Atony

_____ 3. Hematoma

_____ 4. Hematuria

_____ 5. Mastitis

_____ 6. Subinvolution

A. Blood in the urine

B. Lack of pleasure in acts that are normally pleasurable

C. A state in which the uterus fails to complete the involution process after giving birth

D. A lack or an absence of muscle tone of the uterus

E. An infection in the breast tissue

F. A collection of blood in the tissues outside a blood vessel

MATCHING EXERCISE

Postpartum Problems or Complications with Nursing Interventions

_____ 1. Urinary tract infection

_____ 2. Postpartum hemorrhage

_____ 3. Hematoma on the vulva

_____ 4. Engorged breasts

_____ 5. Sore nipples

_____ 6. Thrombophlebitis

_____ 7. Emotionally distressed

_____ 8. Wound infection

_____ 9. Uterine atony

_____ 10. Tender, painful perineum

A. Sitz bath

B. Observe latch-on of the infant

C. Encourage breastfeeding

D. Elevate the legs

E. Obtain a culture to send to the laboratory

F. Massage the uterus and call the health-care provider

G. Provide an ice pack and notify the health-care provider

H. Encourage increased fluid intake

I. Check for distended bladder

J. "You're sad; would you like to talk about it?"

LEARN TO C.U.S.

Short Answer Question

The nurse is caring for a patient who delivered a 10 pound baby 3 hours ago. The nurse notes that the fundus does not stay firm and the patient has soaked a peripad in 10 minutes. The intravenous oxytocin was discontinued 1 hour ago. The nurse will notify the health-care provider using the C.U.S. method of communication. Complete the report.

C: _____

_____

U: _____

_____

S: _____

_____

POST-CONFERENCE ACTIVITY

Short Answer Question

A newly admitted postpartum patient is planning to relinquish her infant for adoption. How can the nurses on the postpartum unit provide therapeutic care and assist her with her plan?

_____

_____

_____

_____

_____

PATIENT TEACHING GUIDELINES

Short Answer Question

Prepare a brief teaching plan on self-care for the adolescent mother.

_____

_____

_____

_____

_____

_____

_____

CONCEPTUAL CORNERSTONE: INFECTION
Short Answer Question

Mary is a 25-year-old G1 P1, 3 days postoperative after a Cesarean birth. She arrived in the Labor and Delivery department in early labor with ruptured membranes and cervical dilation of 3 cm and 75% effaced. Internal fetal monitoring was initiated and she was given IV oxytocin to augment her labor. She progressed slowly over the next 18 hours and was eventually 10 cm dilated, 100% effaced at 0 station. She pushed for 2 hours without progress. At that time, a Cesarean delivery was performed. Today she has a fever of 102.4°F. She complains of lower abdominal pain (not incisional pain) since last evening.

1. What risk factors for infection can you identify?

_____

_____

_____

_____

2. What additional information would you like to know?

_____

_____

_____

_____

3. What actions should the nurse take?

_____

_____

_____

_____

PATIENT TEACHING GUIDELINES: PREVENTING THROMBOSIS (BLOOD CLOTS)

Short Answer Question

Make a list of ways that a patient can prevent blood clots.

1. _____

2. _____

3. _____

4. _____

5. _____

SHORT ANSWER QUESTION

Identify the amount of lochia flow on the pads in Figure 14.1.

Part A: _____

Part B: _____

Part C: _____

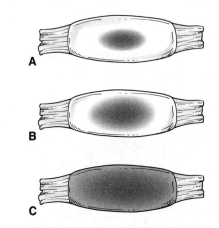

LABEL THE FOLLOWING FIGURE

Identify the location of the fundus immediately after birth and at 24 hours after birth on Figure 14.2.

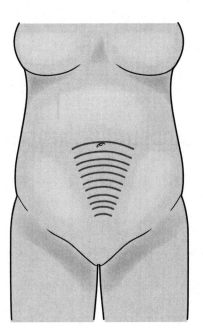

unit FIVE

The Newborn

Physiological and Behavioral Adaptations of the Newborn

Name: _____

Date: _____

Course: _____

Instructor: _____

REVIEW QUESTIONS

1. During labor, the fetal adrenal glands are stimulated to produce dopamine, norepinephrine, and epinephrine. These hormones help the newborn by: (*select all that apply*)
   1. Causing an increase in the level of surfactant in the fetal lungs
   2. Increasing blood flow to the heart, lungs, and brain
   3. Aiding the infant in utilizing brown fat for warmth
   4. Increasing energy
   5. Stimulating white blood cell production
   6. Assisting in establishing passive immunity

2. An infant that is too cold will experience
   1. An increased need for oxygen
   2. A decrease in heart rate
   3. Shivering
   4. Blue hands and feet

3. The purpose of surfactant is to:
   1. Provide energy for the newborn
   2. Provide a heat source for the newborn
   3. Assist the alveoli to remain open
   4. Assist the ductus arteriosus to remain open

4. Which statement indicates that *further teaching is required* when a new mother makes which statement regarding the gastrointestinal transition of her newborn?
   1. "A baby's first stool is a meconium stool."
   2. "Babies at 2-days-old should be able to drink 4 ounces of formula."
   3. "Babies spit up because of an immature sphincter at the stomach and esophagus."
   4. "A baby has no intestinal bacteria at birth."

5. The nurse knows that successful transition of the cardiovascular system has occurred when:
   1. The heart rate is 132 bpm.
   2. The infant has capillary refill time greater than 3 seconds.
   3. The infant's body temperature is 37°C.
   4. The infant's respiratory rate is 66 breaths per minute.

6. Which statement made by a new mother regarding the infant's renal transition indicates *understanding*?
   1. "My 2-day-old infant will have dark yellow urine."
   2. "My 2-day-old infant will have no wet diapers until my breast milk comes in."
   3. "My 2-day-old infant will have at least 2 wet diapers today."
   4. "My 2-day-old infant will have at least 5 wet diapers today."

7. Immediately after birth, a newborn has a heart rate of 58 bpm. The appropriate nursing interventions are: (*select all that apply*)
   1. Call for help.
   2. Place the infant skin-to-skin with the mother.
   3. Dry the infant.
   4. Apply chest compressions.
   5. Provide positive-pressure ventilation.
   6. Inject vitamin K.

8. The nurse notes that a newborn's white blood count is 15,000. The nurse is aware that:
   1. This white blood count indicates a severe infection.
   2. This is a normal white blood count for a newborn.
   3. The doctor must be notified of the white blood count.
   4. This white blood count may indicate a lab error.

9. A newborn is most interested in eating in which wake and sleep state?
   1. Drowsy
   2. Crying
   3. Active alert
   4. Alert

10. The nurse can promote the immune system transition of the newborn by: (*select all that apply*)
    1. Screening visitors for illness
    2. Strict hand washing
    3. Administering vitamin K
    4. Asking the father to wear a mask to cover a cold sore
    5. Bathing the baby as soon as possible

MATCHING EXERCISE

_____ 1. Intestinal bacteria that aid in breaking down food for digestion

_____ 2. The end product of the breakdown of a red blood cell

_____ 3. Hormones produced by the adrenal glands which include dopamine, norepinephrine, and epinephrine

_____ 4. A body temperature below normal

_____ 5. Yellow discoloration of the skin due to the breakdown of red blood cells that are not cleared by the liver

_____ 6. The transfer of body heat to a cooler object, such as a window

_____ 7. Found in term newborns in the scapular area, the thorax, and behind the kidneys, and can be used by the newborn to produce body heat

_____ 8. A mixture of phospholipids and lipoproteins secreted by the lung cells that assists the alveoli to stay open when the newborn begins breathing

_____ 9. The ability of the human body to regulate body temperature at a constant value

_____ 10. Bilirubin that has not been broken down by the liver

A. Thermoregulation

B. Unconjugated bilirubin

C. Hypothermia

D. Radiation

E. Probiotics

F. Jaundice

G. Surfactant

H. Catecholamines

I. Brown fat

J. Bilirubin

SHORT ANSWER QUESTIONS

For Figures 15.1 through 15.4, identify the type of heat loss that can occur and provide a nursing intervention to prevent this type of heat loss.

1.

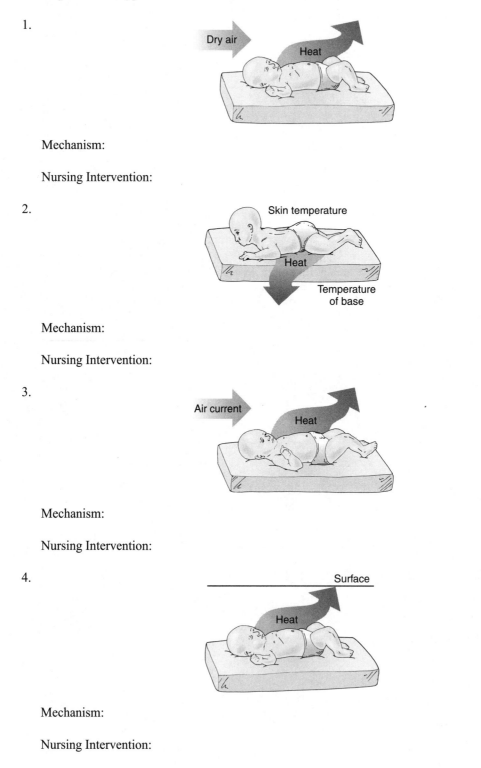

Mechanism:

Nursing Intervention:

2.

Mechanism:

Nursing Intervention:

3.

Mechanism:

Nursing Intervention:

4.

Mechanism:

Nursing Intervention:

💬 LEARN TO C.U.S.

Short Answer Question

The nurse has noticed that a new resident doctor is performing a newborn baby assessment on a 2-hour-old newborn. The resident is very thorough and has had the newborn completely uncovered in a crib for several minutes. The nursery nurse is concerned about thermoregulation for the newborn and uses the C.U.S. method to discuss it with the resident.

Write out an appropriate discussion using the C.U.S. method.

_____

_____

_____

CIRCULATION CHANGES

Short Answer Questions

Identify the areas of the circulatory system in Figure 15.5 that change when the fetus transitions to extra uterine life.

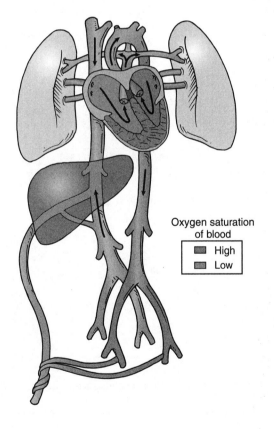

Oxygen saturation
of blood

■ High
■ Low

1.

2.

3.

SHORT ANSWER QUESTIONS

1. What mechanical mechanism assists with initiation of breathing?

   _____

   _____

2. What are the chemical initiators of breathing?

   _____

3. After birth, which two changes occur in the circulatory system to increase blood flow to the lungs?

   _____

   _____

4. What changes occur in the circulation to increase blood flow to the newborn's liver after birth?

   _____

   _____

5. What is physiologic jaundice?

   _____

   _____

6. What vitamin affects blood clotting?

   _____

7. What behaviors indicate the newborn is in the drowsy state?

   _____

   _____

8. What behaviors indicate that the newborn is in the active alert state?

   _____

   _____

   _____

9. If the newborn's heart rate is less than 60 bpm, what should the nurse do?

   _____

   _____

10. What is the appropriate action for the nurse to promote during the first period of reactivity?

   _____

   _____

PATIENT TEACHING GUIDELINES

Short Answer Question

Prepare a short patient teaching guideline regarding normal physiologic jaundice for parents.

_____

_____

_____

THERAPEUTIC COMMUNICATION

Short Answer Questions

A mother calls the postpartum unit and is concerned about the behavior of her 5-day-old infant. Fill in a therapeutic response to the mother's questions.

1. Mother: "I don't know what to do . . . My baby has been crying a lot this evening."

   Nurse: _____

2. Mother: "How can I know what my baby wants?"

   Nurse: _____

3. Mother: "Should I try to wake my baby up for feedings?"

   Nurse: _____

4. Mother: "Sometimes he gets all fussy and isn't happy even if I try to nurse him."

   Nurse: _____

SAFETY STAT!

Short Answer Question

List three safety issues that can be identified from this chapter on newborn transition after birth.

1. _____

2. _____

3. _____

FILL-IN-THE-BLANK QUESTION

Fill in the blanks to describe the process of removal of bilirubin from the body.

The _____ changes the yellow pigment from the breakdown of the red blood cell into a water-soluble pigment that can be excreted by the body. The removal of _____ _____ begins when _____ remove old red blood cells from the circulation. As the red blood cells break down, _____, the oxygen-carrying component of hemoglobin is broken down into iron, carbon monoxide, and biliverdin. The biliverdin is broken down further into _____. The bilirubin attaches to _____ in the blood and travels to the _____. In the _____, an enzyme called glucuronyl transferese acts upon the bilirubin to change it into a water-soluble pigment called _____ _____ _____ that is excreted into the common duct and duodenum. Once the direct bilirubin is in the intestine, the normal intestinal flora reduces the _____ _____ into _____ and stercolinogen. These are excreted mainly in the stool, causing the yellowish brown color of the stool, and a small amount is excreted in the urine.

Assessment and Care of the Newborn

Name: _____

Date: _____

Course: _____

Instructor: _____

REVIEW QUESTIONS

1. A mother is holding her 6-hour-old infant. She makes the statement, "He has such a cone head!" The best response by the nurse is:
   1. "That is called molding and it will go away in about 1 month."
   2. "That is called molding and it will go away in just a few days."
   3. "That is called molding and we need to report it to the pediatrician."
   4. "That is called molding and it tends to be common in some families."

2. The nurse is about to elicit the rooting reflex. Which of the following responses should the nurse expect to see?
   1. When the baby is suddenly startled, the newborn's arms straighten outward and the knees flex.
   2. When the baby is placed on his back with the head turned to one side, the arm on that side extends out.
   3. When the cheek of the baby is touched lightly, the baby turns toward the side that was touched.
   4. When the lateral aspect of the baby's foot is stroked, the toes extend and fan outward.

3. A nurse is assessing a newborn on admission to the nursery. The nurse would report which of the following assessment findings?
   1. Retractions of the chest when breathing
   2. Caput succedaneum
   3. Lanugo
   4. Purple patches on the buttocks

4. The nurse is careful to wear gloves when caring for a newborn who has not been bathed for the first time. Which of the following is the rationale for this action?
   1. The baby is at increased risk of infection right after birth and needs to be protected.
   2. The baby's skin is delicate and the nurse could cause a rash when holding the newborn.
   3. The amniotic fluid may contain viruses.
   4. The vernix caseosa can be irritating to the nurse's hands.

5. The nurse is teaching the parents about circumcision care. Which of the following should be included in the teaching plan? (*select all that apply*)
   1. Use a soft cloth to gently remove the yellow crust that will form around the circumcision site.
   2. Give a sponge bath until the circumcision is healed and the Plasti-bell falls off if used.
   3. Keep the penis as dry as possible.
   4. A small amount of blood-tinged drainage may be noticed right after the procedure.
   5. Do not call the doctor until the baby has a fever greater than 102°F (38.9°C) axillary.

6. A new mother asks the nurse how to care for the umbilical cord until it falls off. The nurse should advise the new mother to:
   1. Clean the cord with hydrogen peroxide twice a day.
   2. Give a tub bath daily to keep the cord moist.
   3. Call the doctor when it falls off.
   4. Fold the diaper below the cord to expose it to air.

7. A nurse is providing guidance about newborn sleeping. Which of the following should be included? (*select all that apply*)
   1. A newborn will sleep better lying on the tummy in a crib near the parents.
   2. A newborn should be covered with several blankets in order to stay warm.
   3. A newborn should be placed on the back in a crib near the parents.
   4. A newborn should be dressed in layers for warmth.
   5. A newborn will sleep better lying on the back in the parent's bed.

8. A mother asks the nurse why her baby has a "bump" on one side of the head. The nurse notes that the bump covers the left parietal bone but does not cross the suture lines of the skull. The nurse explains to the mother that the "bump" is:
   1. Caused by the position the baby preferred in the uterus before birth
   2. Molding of the skull as the baby went through the pelvis
   3. Swelling due to the rupture of blood vessels during pushing and delivery
   4. Swelling due to the pressure of the head going through the birth canal

9. During an initial assessment, the nurse places a clean-gloved finger into the newborn's mouth. The nurse is assessing for: (*select all that apply*)
   1. To see if the newborn has an intact palate
   2. The color of the mucous membranes
   3. The symmetry of the lips
   4. The suck reflex
   5. The rooting reflex

10. The nurse notices the new father holding the newborn and not supporting the infant's head. The nurse should:
    1. Immediately take the newborn from the father
    2. Ask to hold the infant and then demonstrate the correct way to hold the infant
    3. Quietly tell the mother that she should not let the father hold the infant
    4. Bring an infant safety DVD to the bedside and require the father to watch it

MATCHING EXERCISE
Newborn Reflexes

_____ 1. The newborn turns the mouth to the same side of the cheek that was stroked.

_____ 2. In response to a sudden movement, the newborn abducts the extremities and places the index finger and thumb into a "C" shape.

_____ 3. The newborn simulates walking when held in an upright position and the soles of the feet touch a firm surface.

_____ 4. A cough in response to stimulation of the posterior oral cavity.

_____ 5. The newborn flexes the big toe when the foot is stroked along the sole of the foot from the heel to the head of the fifth metatarsal.

_____ 6. In a supine position, if the head is turned to one side, the newborn will extend the arm and leg on that side and flex the arm and leg on the other side.

_____ 7. The newborn wraps the fingers around the examiner's finger.

_____ 8. The newborn uses the tongue to push foreign objects out of the mouth.

_____ 9. The newborn's toes curl downward in response to pressure applied to the sole of the foot at the base of the toes.

A. Moro
B. Gag
C. Babinski
D. Plantar
E. Tonic neck
F. Extrusion
G. Stepping
H. Palmar
I. Rooting

FILL-IN-THE-BLANK QUESTIONS

1. Dermal melanosis is also known as a _____ _____.

2. The medical term for the newborn's "soft spot" is _____.

3. _____ are sebaceous glands that are occluded with keratin usually located on the chin, nose, and cheeks of the newborn.

4. A _____ _____, also known as *stork bites*, is caused by capillary malformations in the skin.

5. Enlarged breasts in the newborn are known as _____.

6. A newborn born after 42 weeks gestation is called _____.

7. Blood-tinged mucous found in the female infant's diaper is known as _____.

8. Blue hands and feet of the newborn are known as _____.

9. A newborn is having difficulty breathing, and the nurse notices that the skin pulls in around the ribs and sternum. This is known as _____.

10. The medical term for a port-wine birthmark is _____ _____.

TRUE OR FALSE QUESTIONS

1. _____ An absence of hand and foot creases could indicate a preterm infant.

2. _____ Lanugo is a white protective coating on the skin of the newborn.

3. _____ A strawberry hemangioma will usually fade without medical interventions.

4. _____ Acne neonatorum are clogged hair follicles or pores in the skin.

5. _____ Gynecomastia should be reported immediately to the health-care provider.

6. _____ See-saw chest movements and retraction of the skin around the ribs and sternum are normal characteristics of the newborn breathing pattern.

7. _____ When the nurse listens to the newborn's heart, the nurse should first listen for the normal S1 and S2 heart sounds.

8. _____ The nurse should report a heart rate less than 110 bpm or greater than 160 bpm at rest.

9. _____ The meconium stool should be passed within 2 hours of birth.

10. _____ Asymmetrical thigh creases are expected in the newborn for 24 hours.

11. _____ A gestational age assessment should be completed on preterm and post-term newborns.

12. _____ Early identification of hearing problems with early treatment can prevent severe speech problems for a child.

13. _____ Placing the baby on the stomach for a few minutes each day can prevent flat spots on the head.

14. _____ A negative Ortolani exam indicates that the hips are normal.

15. _____ Epstein pearls are little teeth found in the mouth of the newborn.

SAFETY *STAT!*

Shade the areas where a nurse can safely perform a newborn heel stick (Fig. 16.1).

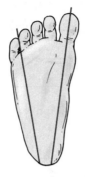

POST-CONFERENCE ACTIVITY

Short Answer Questions

Prepare a list of "dos and don'ts" appropriate for first time parents leaving the hospital with their newborn.

_____

_____

_____

_____

_____

_____

_____

_____

_____

_____

_____

THERAPEUTIC COMMUNICATION

Short-Answer Questions

Write a therapeutic response to the following situations.

1. The nurse is trying to teach a new mother about basic infant care. She does not seem to be able to focus on the teaching and looks to be on the verge of tears.

_____

_____

2. A patient states, "My mother says that babies are supposed to sleep on their stomachs so that they won't choke if they spit up during sleep."

_____

_____

3. A patient states, "I can't decide about circumcision. I really don't know what to do!"

_____

_____

4. A patient is breastfeeding her newborn and states, "I didn't realize that babies have to eat so often!"

_____

_____

5. A patient that is being discharged states, "I forgot what you said about taking care of his umbilical cord. I'm going to be a terrible mother."

_____

_____

6. A patient confides to the nurse that she does not have a crib for her newborn.

_____

_____

_____

7. A patient states to the nurse, "Would it be okay if I put a tiny little dab of acne medication on my baby's nose? Those white heads are so awful."

_____

_____

8. During discharge teaching about bathing the baby, the mother asks, "Can't I just bathe him with my 2-year-old? It would save a lot of time."

_____

_____

LEARN TO C.U.S.

Short Answer Question

A nurse is assessing a 2-hour-old post-term newborn and notices that the respiratory rate is 60, the heart rate is 182, there are retractions of the skin around the sternum, and the newborn has a blue tint around the lips.

The nurse calls the health-care provider using the C.U.S. method of communication.

_____

_____

_____

ILLUSTRATION EXERCISE

Identify the diagrams of head conditions that may be observed in the newborn.

1. Figure 16.2: _____

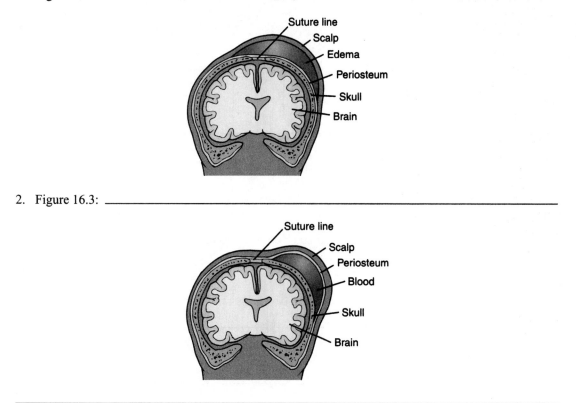

2. Figure 16.3: _____

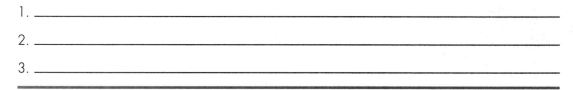

SAFETY *STAT!*

Short Answer Questions

List at least three signs of complications after a circumcision.

1. _____

2. _____

3. _____

TABLE COMPLETION
Normal Newborn Vital Signs

| Temperature |
| Heart Rate |
| Respiratory Rate |
| Blood Pressure |

SAFETY *STAT!*

Short Answer Questions

List warning signs observed during physical assessment that should be immediately reported.

1. _____

2. _____

3. _____

4. _____

5. _____

6. _____

7. _____

8. _____

Newborn Nutrition

Name: _____

Date: _____

Course: _____

Instructor: _____

REVIEW QUESTIONS

1. A multipara patient on the postpartum unit states, "I quit breastfeeding with my first baby because I did not have enough milk. I wish I could breastfeed this baby." The best response by the nurse is:
   1. "More frequent nursing will increase your milk supply."
   2. "Not everyone can nurse a baby."
   3. "I wouldn't worry about it."
   4. "I am sure your baby did fine with formula."

2. A new mother is learning to breastfeed. She asks the nurse to tell her if enough of her breast is in the baby's mouth. The nurse knows that the correct mouth position for the breastfeeding infant is:
   1. Lips are positioned around the nipple only.
   2. The mouth is open wide with most or all of the areola inside the mouth.
   3. The lips are turned in and the infant makes a "clicking" sound when suckling.
   4. The top lip is turned out and the bottom lip is turned inward toward the breast.

3. A woman develops breast engorgement on her fourth postpartum day. Her breasts are so engorged that she cannot get the baby to latch-on correctly. She calls the hospital nursery for support. The nurse should advise the patient to:
   1. Bottle feed the baby and let her breasts rest.
   2. Reduce her fluid intake for 24 hours.
   3. Apply heat to the breasts; express enough milk to soften the breast.
   4. Feed the baby every hour for the next 24 hours.

4. Breastfeeding is contraindicated for women who: (*select all that apply*)
   1. Are HIV-positive.
   2. Take Tylenol for a headache.
   3. Are addicted to heroin.
   4. Are underweight.
   5. Drink one beer with pizza once a month.

5. The lactation consultant calls the home of a new breastfeeding woman who has a 4-day-old infant. The mother reports that she has been breastfeeding every 4 hours and the baby has had only two wet diapers today. The nurse should advise the woman to:
   1. Bring the baby to the hospital immediately.
   2. Maintain the breastfeeding schedule.
   3. Feed the baby every 2 to 2½ hours.
   4. Give the baby a water bottle.

6. When planning patient instructions on breastfeeding, the nurse includes the following instructions related to milk supply:
   1. Her breast size is a very important influence on milk supply.
   2. The mother's body weight influences milk supply.
   3. The amount of nipple stimulation and the time the baby nurses influence milk supply.
   4. The mother's fluid intake influences milk supply.

7. When teaching the parents about preparing infant formula, it is important to include which instruction?
   1. For powdered and concentrated formula, adjust the amount of water added based on the infant's weight-gain pattern.
   2. Make sure the infant takes all the formula in the bottle.
   3. Add any leftover formula from a feeding to the bottle for the next feeding.
   4. Wash the formula containers when you bring them home from the store.

8. Newborn cues that the infant will be responsive to breastfeeding include: (*select all that apply*)
   1. Putting the hand in the mouth
   2. Crying loudly
   3. Passing gas
   4. Rooting reflex
   5. Tonic neck reflex

9. The nurse is observing a new mother bottle feed her newborn. The nurse notes good bottle feeding technique after observing: (*select all that apply*)
   1. The mother holds the infant close with the head elevated.
   2. The mother enlarged the hole in the nipple to allow faster formula flow.
   3. The mother keeps the nipple full of formula.
   4. The mother stops and burps the baby periodically.

10. The nurse is observing a new mother position her newborn for breastfeeding. The nurse notes good breastfeeding positioning after observing: (*select all that apply*)
    1. The mother supports her breast with her fingers underneath and thumb on top.
    2. The mother checks for placement of the newborn tongue before feeding.
    3. The mother leans over to bring her breast toward the baby.
    4. The infant's jaws are compressing the nipple.

FILL-IN-THE-BLANK QUESTIONS

1. The first substance produced by the breast before mature milk is made is called

   _____.

2. A(n) _____ is a protein that functions as an antibody and is present in breast milk.

3. The process of the body producing milk is called _____.

4. The hormone responsible for milk production is called _____.

5. The milk produced and stored between breastfeeding sessions is called

   _____.

6. The American Academy of Pediatrics recommends exclusive _____ for the first 6 months of age.

7. Concentrated infant formula should be diluted with _____.

8. A bottle should never be warmed in the _____.

9. A _____ _____ may need to assist a woman with flat or inverted nipples with establishing breastfeeding.

TABLE COMPLETION

Complete the following table on breastfeeding problems and nursing interventions.

Breastfeeding Problem	Nursing Interventions
Sore nipples	
Nipple confusion	
Low milk supply	
Engorgement	
Flat or inverted nipples	

TRUE OR FALSE QUESTIONS

1. _____ The World Health Organization suggests that babies be breastfed for 2 years.

2. _____ A baby under the age of 6 months does not require water supplements.

3. _____ Prolactin stimulates milk production.

4. _____ Most medications do not pass through breastmilk.

5. _____ The breastfeeding mother should wash her breasts before each feeding.

6. _____ The mother's hand should be in the "C" position as she supports her breast during latch-on.

7. _____ A 6-day-old infant should have 2 to 3 wet diapers per day.

8. _____ Ready-to-feed formula should not be diluted with water.

9. _____ A bottle that has been sitting out of the refrigerator for 20 minutes is safe to use.

10. _____ Cow's milk has a high level of iron and protein.

POST-CONFERENCE ACTIVITY

Search the nursing literature for articles related to breastfeeding. Summarize the main points and discuss how a health-care professional can use the article's information to improve health care.

CONCEPTUAL CORNERSTONE

Discuss the potential negative effects of giving an infant cow's milk before 1 year of age.

CULTURAL CONSIDERATIONS

Interview a postpartum patient during clinical about her reasons for choosing her method of feeding. Were any of the reasons based on cultural influences?

LEARN TO C.U.S.

A couple brings their 3-year-old child to the emergency department because he has croup and ear pain. They have brought along their 2-month-old infant. While waiting for the physician, the nurse notes that the parents have propped the bottle for the infant while dealing with their fussy 3-year-old. Write out a possible conversation with the parents using the C.U.S. method of communication to address the issue with the parents.

C: _____

U: _____

S: _____

NURSING CARE PLAN

Jennifer is a new mother on the postpartum unit. She delivered her baby 36 hours ago. During the assessment at the beginning of the shift, the nurse notes that Jennifer has sore nipples and states that it is "very painful to breastfeed. It makes me want to cry." Prepare an appropriate care plan for Jennifer.

Newborn at Risk: Conditions Present at Birth

Name: _____

Date: _____

Course: _____

Instructor: _____

MATCHING EXERCISE

_____ 1. Extremely premature

_____ 2. Very premature

_____ 3. Moderately premature

_____ 4. Late preterm

_____ 5. Early-term

_____ 6. Full-term

_____ 7. Late-term

_____ 8. Post-term

A. Born between 37 weeks, 6 days and 38 weeks, 6 days

B. Born between 34 and 37 weeks gestation

C. Born between 39 weeks and 40 weeks, 6 days

D. Born less than 28 weeks gestation

E. Born less than 32 weeks gestation

F. Born between 41 weeks and 41 weeks, 6 days

G. Born 42 weeks or beyond

H. Born less than 34 weeks gestation

REVIEW QUESTIONS

1. Part of the medical treatment for necrotizing enterocolitis includes is:
   1. Antibiotics
   2. High-calorie formula
   3. Caffeine
   4. Decreased stimulation

2. The nurse has been teaching the mother about apnea of prematurity. Which statement indicates that the mother *understands* the teaching?
   1. "My baby will have apnea problems until she is a toddler."
   2. "There are no medications to stimulate her breathing."
   3. "She will outgrow the apnea as her brain and lungs mature."
   4. "I must shake her when the alarm goes off."

3. Possible long-term complications of prenatal drug exposure include: (*select all that apply*)
   1. Hyperactivity
   2. Poor language development
   3. Polycythemia
   4. Necrotizing enterocolitis
   5. Learning disabilities

4. A physical characteristic of a preterm baby is:
   1. Lack of ear cartilage
   2. Many sole creases
   3. No vernix
   4. Hypertonia

5. A possible complication for a large-for-gestational-age newborn is:
   1. Jaundice
   2. Poor feeding
   3. Enterocolitis
   4. Birth injuries

6. A premature newborn of 32 weeks has been admitted to the nursery. A priority intervention for this newborn is:
   1. Notifying the neonatologist
   2. Performing a gestational age assessment
   3. Providing for warmth
   4. Administering vitamin K

7. Polycythemia develops in the infant of a diabetic mother because:
   1. The fetus is adapting to hypoxia.
   2. The mother is anemic.
   3. Too much glucose is crossing the placenta.
   4. The mother is Rh-negative.

8. A possible complication of polycythemia is:
   1. Low blood sugar
   2. Irritability
   3. Jaundice
   4. Dehydration

9. A student nurse asks the Neonatal Intensive Care Unit (NICU) nurse when to expect withdrawal symptoms for the newborn exposed to heroin. The nurse's response is
   1. 6 to 12 hours
   2. 12 to 24 hours
   3. 24 to 72 hours
   4. 72 to 96 hours

10. The nurse observes the student nurse holding a drug-exposed newborn in the nursery. The nurse knows that the student nurse is knowledgeable about the care of a drug-exposed baby when the nurse sees the student nurse:
    1. Laughing loudly while holding the newborn.
    2. Holding the newborn securely facing outward from her body.
    3. Uncovering the complete body all at one time for an assessment.
    4. Placing the crib in the center of the nursery.

SHORT ANSWER QUESTIONS

1. Zidovudine is a drug used for _____.

2. For the premature newborn, the drug of choice to treat apnea of prematurity is

   _____.

3. Intrauterine growth restriction is due to _____.

4. List five possible causes of a small-for-gestational-age newborn.
   1.
   2.
   3.
   4.
   5.

FILL-IN-THE-BLANK QUESTIONS

1. _____ _____ _____ is a
   group of similar behavioral and physiological symptoms in the neonate caused by withdrawal from
   pharmacological agents.

2. A potential complication for the premature newborn related to the eyes is

   _____ _____.

3. Heavy smokers can give birth to a _____ or a _____
   newborn.

4. _____ may be administered to the newborn to control withdrawal seizures.

5. A _____ _____ may occur during a
   vaginal delivery of a large-for-gestational-age fetus.

6. Newborns can get low blood sugar or hypoglycemia because of lack of stored

   _____ in the liver.

TRUE OR FALSE QUESTIONS

1. _____ Intraventricular hemorrhage is a common complication of small-for-gestational-age newborns.

2. _____ Premature infants are at risk for anemia.

3. _____ Hypertension in pregnancy is a risk factor for a potential problem in the newborn.

4. _____ Transmission of HIV from the mother to the fetus cannot be prevented by taking antiretroviral
   medication during pregnancy.

5. _____ A sign of caffeine withdrawal in the newborn is diarrhea.

6. _____ If a pregnant woman goes overdue, there is a chance that the placenta may not be functioning
   properly to support the infant.

7. _____ Only the nurses should wear gloves when holding an HIV-exposed infant.

8. _____ Drug-exposed newborns enjoy stimulation.

9. _____ The onset of withdrawal symptoms depends upon the drug and the timing of the last ingestion
   or use by the mother.

10. _____ The infant of a diabetic mother is usually macrosomic.

MATCHING EXERCISE

_____ 1. Apnea

_____ 2. Hematochezia

_____ 3. Hyperinsulinemia

_____ 4. Hypoglycemia

_____ 5. Hypomagnesemia

_____ 6. Hypoxia

_____ 7. Macrosomia

_____ 8. Necrosis

_____ 9. Polycythemia

_____ 10. Necrotizing
    enterocolitis

A. A disease of premature infants characterized by damage to the intestinal tract mucosa.

B. The passage of bright red fresh blood in the stool.

C. Cessation of breathing for more than 20 seconds.

D. An excess of red blood cells.

E. A decrease in oxygen supply to the tissues.

F. A plasma glucose level of less than 30 mg/dL in the first 24 hours of life.

G. The death of cells, tissues, or organs.

H. A condition of excess insulin circulating in the blood.

I. Birth weight greater than 4000 g or above the 90th percentile for gestational age.

J. Low levels of magnesium in the blood.

 DRUG FACTS: CALCULATION QUESTIONS

Short Answer Questions

Calculate the correct dosage for each of these medications discussed in the text.

1. Doctor's order: Administer phenobarbital 3 mg/kg/day PO divided twice a day. Calculate the single dose for the newborn that weighs 3 kg.

2. Doctor's order: Administer Zidovudine 4 mg/kg PO in one dose to a newborn that weighs 2.8 kg. The medication strength is 50 mg/5mL. How many milliliters will you administer?

3. Doctor's order: Administer nevirapine 12 mg/kg in one dose to a newborn that weighs 2 kg. The medication strength is 50 mg/mL. How many milligrams will you administer?

4. Doctor's order: Administer caffeine 5 mg/kg PO in one dose to a 28-week-old premature newborn that weighs 1.2 kg. The medication strength is 20 mg/mL. How many milliliters will you administer?

THERAPEUTIC COMMUNICATION: REVIEW QUESTIONS

1. A mother of a 35 week gestation newborn is in the NICU holding her baby. She remarks to the nurse, "I wish my baby weighed 11 pounds like my sister's baby weighed. Then she wouldn't have any problems."

   Select the answer that is the most therapeutic.

   1. "A large baby can have plenty of problems, too."
   2. "Don't worry, your baby will be fine."
   3. "What problems are you most concerned about?"
   4. "You should be happy that she made it."

2. The mother states, "She is so skinny."
   Select the answer that is most therapeutic.
   1. "She will continue to grow and will gain weight."
   2. "Girls always want to be skinny."
   3. "There's nothing wrong with being skinny."
   4. "Being skinny is the least of her problems."
3. The nurse overhears the mother say, "When I get her home, I can add cereal to her diet and put weight on her faster."
   Select the most therapeutic response.
   1. "That would not be a good idea, at all!"
   2. "You need to ask your doctor about that."
   3. "That's a good idea."
   4. "Her gastrointestinal system is immature. It's too early to introduce baby cereal".

PATIENT TEACHING GUIDELINES

Short Answer Questions

Prepare brief patient teaching for a group of insulin-dependent diabetic women that are planning to become pregnant.

_____

_____

_____

_____

_____

LEARN TO C.U.S.

Short Answer Question

A patient in labor and delivery admits to a history of drug use. She did not have adequate prenatal care. She confides to the nurse that she is concerned because her partner, the baby's father is an IV drug user and is HIV-positive. The nurse notifies the doctor using the C.U.S. method of communication.

C: _____

U: _____

S: _____

SAFETY STAT!

Short Answer Question

A patient that admits to the use of Vicodin daily during her pregnancy. In preparation for the delivery, list safety issues that should be addressed.

_____

_____

Newborn at Risk: Birth-Related Stressors

Name: _____

Date: _____

Course: _____

Instructor: _____

REVIEW QUESTIONS

1. There are four babies in the nursery. The nurse contacts the physician to see the baby who exhibits:
   1. Acrocyanosis
   2. Blood glucose of 40 mg/dL
   3. Tachypnea
   4. Axillary temperature of 98.2°F (36.8°C)

2. A baby is receiving phototherapy for jaundice. The nurse is providing safe care when:
   1. The infant is wrapped in a warm blanket.
   2. The infant is dressed in a t-shirt and diaper.
   3. The infant is removed from the light source for 5 minutes every hour.
   4. The infant's eyes are covered with eye pads.

3. The nurse notes that a term newborn has a large cephalohematoma and a bruise on the face from forceps. The nurse should monitor the baby carefully for which of the following?
   1. Hypoglycemia
   2. Hyperbilirubinemia
   3. Hypothermia
   4. Hypercapnia

4. A post-term baby was admitted to the nursery. At delivery, thick green meconium fluid was noted and his skin has a greenish tint. Which of the following actions should the nurse do *first?*
   1. Bathe the baby to remove the meconium from the skin.
   2. Begin a head-to-toe assessment.
   3. Begin with a respiratory assessment.
   4. Administer the newborn vitamin K.

5. A 10 lb, 6 oz baby boy was delivered and the birth was complicated by a shoulder dystocia. Which birth injury is *most likely* for this newborn? (*select all that apply*)
    1. Brachial plexus injury
    2. Spinal cord injury
    3. Fractured clavicle
    4. Kernicterus
    5. Fractured radius

6. A baby was just born before the mother could receive her antibiotics for group B streptococcus. Which of the following complications may occur for this newborn?
    1. Hyperbilirubinemia
    2. Neonatal sepsis
    3. Hypoglycemia
    4. Hypercapnia

7. The nurse is auscultating the heart sounds of a term newborn that was just delivered. The nurse notes that the baby is cyanotic despite administering oxygen and the nurse can hear a loud heart murmur. The nurse notifies the pediatrician because the nurse suspects:
    1. Neonatal sepsis
    2. Hypoglycemia
    3. Meconium aspiration syndrome
    4. Persistent pulmonary hypertension

8. Which of the following mechanisms are used when the newborn's body tries to raise the body temperature? (*select all that apply*)
    1. Peripheral vasoconstriction causes the blood to go to the core of the body to warm major organs.
    2. The heme from red blood cells binds with albumin for excretion.
    3. The foramen ovale remains open and shunts blood away from the lungs.
    4. Brown fat is metabolized to warm the blood in the core.

9. A mother brings her 5-day-old baby to the lactation clinic for help with breastfeeding. The nurse notes that the infant is lethargic, has a temperature of 95.5°F (35.3°C), is eating poorly, and has cool clammy skin. The nurse instructs the mother to:
    1. Take the newborn to the emergency room now.
    2. Feed the baby more often.
    3. Dress the baby in warmer clothes.
    4. Start bottle feeding.

10. The nurse checks the blood sugar on a term newborn that is 10 hours old. The reading on the glucometer is 28 mg/dL. The nurse should:
    1. Recheck in 1 hour and if still 28 mg/dL, call the health-care provider.
    2. Take the baby to the mother for breastfeeding.
    3. Notify the health-care provider immediately.
    4. Administer intravenous glucose.

MATCHING EXERCISE

_____ 1. Rapid breathing

_____ 2. Excessive carbon dioxide in the blood stream

_____ 3. Brain dysfunction caused by excessive bilirubin

_____ 4. No oxygen reaching cells

_____ 5. Insufficient oxygen reaching the cells

_____ 6. Labored or difficult breathing

_____ 7. The amount of insulin in the blood is higher than normal.

_____ 8. Collapse of a lung

A. Anoxia

B. Dyspnea

C. Hypercapnia

D. Hyperinsulinism

E. Hypoxia

F. Kernicterus

G. Pneumothorax

H. Tachypnea

SHORT ANSWER QUESTIONS

1. What are the signs of hypoglycemia?

_____

_____

2. List three nursing interventions for providing family-centered care in the Neonatal Intensive Care Unit (NICU)?

_____

_____

_____

3. List three risk factors for hyperbilirubinemia?

_____

_____

_____

4. Write a nursing diagnosis for a newborn with hyperbilirubinemia.

_____

5. List three nursing interventions for a newborn undergoing phototherapy.

_____

_____

_____

6. Why do nurses decrease stimulation for a sick neonate?

_____

7. A premature baby is born and is developing cold stress. List appropriate nursing interventions to manage cold stress.

_____

_____

_____

8. List the health-care team members that may be involved in the care of an infant with a brachial plexus injury.

_____

_____

_____

9. Write a nursing diagnosis for the infant with meconium aspiration syndrome.

_____

10. What is pathologic jaundice? How does it differ from physiologic jaundice?

_____

POST-CONFERENCE ACTIVITIES

1. Research resources available for parents of babies in the NICU. The resources could be for emotional support such as support groups or monetary support for the cost of care in the NICU.

2. Briefly interview a nurse who works in the NICU and inquire about the nurse's career path and education required for becoming a nurse in the NICU. Share your findings at post-conference.

PATIENT TEACHING GUIDELINES

Short Answer Question

A 48-hour-old newborn is being discharged from the newborn nursery. The nurse is aware that the newborn had no complications from birth and has been stable and breastfeeding well. The nurse notices that the newborn's face is slightly yellow. What discharge instructions should the nurse give the parents?

_____

_____

_____

LEARN TO C.U.S.

Short Answer Question

A newborn in the nursery has tachypnea and requires oxygen to keep the O_2 saturation levels above 93%. The physician diagnosed the newborn with transient tachypnea. The nurse notes that the tachypnea is getting worse and the respiratory rate is now 60 beats per minute with grunting, flaring, and chest retractions. The nurse is concerned and communicates with the doctor using the C.U.S. method. Write out the communication using the C.U.S. method.

C: _____

U: _____

S: _____

THERAPEUTIC COMMUNICATION

Short Answer Question

A nurse in the NICU observes a mother standing at the bedside of her baby. The baby has a chest tube inserted due to a pneumothorax from a meconium aspiration. The mother is crying. Write a therapeutic opening sentence for communicating with the mother.

_____

The mother states, "I feel so overwhelmed. This is not what I planned."

The nurse answers: _____

The mother states, "I feel so guilty. I must have done something wrong."

The nurse answers: _____

The mother states, "Do you think he will be alright?"

The nurse answers: _____

 ## CULTURAL CONSIDERATIONS

Short Answer Question

Consider your own cultural or religious background and in a few sentences describe how you or your family would handle a crisis, such as a sick newborn.

_____

_____

_____

PATIENT TEACHING GUIDELINES

Short Answer Question

You need to briefly explain to a new mother why her post-term, large baby needs to have his blood sugar monitored. Write your explanation for the mother here.

_____

_____

_____

NEONATAL SEPSIS

Concept Map Completion

Neonatal sepsis can be caused by bacteria or virus but the symptoms, medical management, and nursing interventions are similar regardless of the cause. Using your textbook as a guide, complete the concept map (Fig. 19.1) about neonatal sepsis, beginning with listing in the boxes, the infective agents, either viral or bacterial, list the symptoms, and then move on to medical management, medications, and nursing interventions.

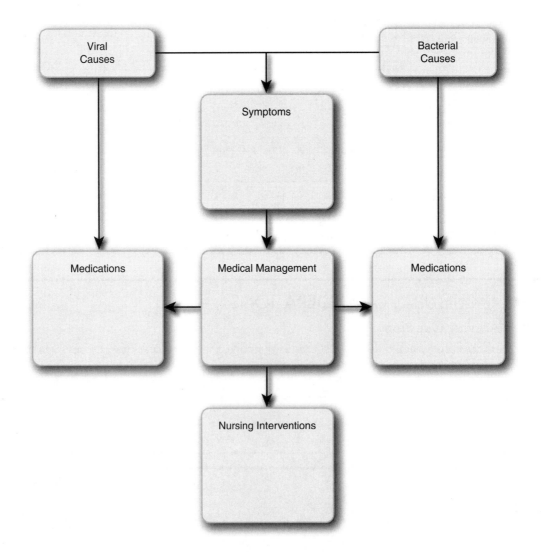

unit SIX

Growth and Development

Introduction to Pediatric Nursing

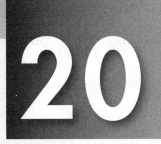

20

Name: _____

Date: _____

Course: _____

Instructor: _____

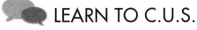 **LEARN TO C.U.S.**

Short Answer Question

Maintaining safety is an important responsibility of the pediatric health-care team. On day three of the admission of a family of twin middle school boys, you notice the room is rearranged to have the bed against the windows, clutter is all over the floor, the boys are often roaming the halls without their parents, and there is evidence that the boys are playing with the charting mobile computers in the room meant only for the health-care team. How might you use the Learn to C.U.S. method of communication to address the children and their parents?

C: _____

U: _____

S: _____

THERAPEUTIC COMMUNICATION

Short Answer Question

The single mother of an 11-month-old hospitalized infant is crying incessantly as the mother is preparing to leave to go to work for the day. As the mother is crying she tells the nurse how difficult it is to leave her infant in the hospital. What is a therapeutic communication statement that can be made to reassure the mother?

_____

_____

_____

CULTURAL CONSIDERATIONS

Short Answer Questions

Issues related to "new morbidity" are especially concerning for families living in geographic areas of low income. Violence, crowded living conditions, and unsafe living arrangements can all contribute to issues of new morbidity. Define the concept of "New Morbidity" and list three concerns related to this term:

1. Definition:

   _____

   _____

2. Three concerns:

   1. _____

   2. _____

   3. _____

SAFETY *STAT!*

True or False Questions

1. _____ The term *new morbidity* is used to describe the most recently experienced pathologies diagnosed in the pediatric population.

2. _____ The development stage of the toddler spans from 11 months of age through the third birthday.

3. _____ Two important concepts of the philosophy of family-centered care are enabling and empowerment.

4. _____ There are concerns about adult medical surgical nurses caring for pediatric patients in health-care institutions that do not provide pediatric beds. Three concerns are pediatric-specific skills; neonatal, infant, and child CPR; and medication dosage calculations.

SAFETY *STAT!*

Short Answer Question

It is important for a pediatric nurse to be aware of the concerns surrounding medication errors. There are four main areas of medication errors found in pediatrics. List the four:

1. _____

2. _____

3. _____

4. _____

TEAM WORKS

Fill-in-the-Blank Question

The philosophy of family-centered care recognizes the family as the _____ in the child's life and that all members of the family are indeed affected by the illness, injury, or hospitalization that the child is experiencing. Furthermore, the foundation of family-centered care includes the need to provide support based on respect, _____, the _____ _____ _____, and the _____ _____ _____.

PATIENT TEACHING GUIDELINES

Matching Exercise

Match the following child temperament behaviors with the title of the type of temperament:

_____ 1. Active, feisty, or difficult children

_____ 2. Slow-to-warm-up or cautious children

_____ 3. Easy children who demonstrate flexibility

A. Tend to demonstrate the need for more time to accept new situations, new activities, and new social interactions. They may display a more moody temperament with inactivity before acceptance. These children may appear to withdraw or have trouble with new people and new situations.

B. Tend to demonstrate more intense reactions to new situations and may fight against change or react with a sense of negative withdrawal. These children may be easily upset by commotion and demonstrate difficult feeding, sleeping, and social behaviors.

C. Tend to demonstrate behaviors that are predictable or regular and will generally approach new situations, people, and circumstances with a positive attitude. Easy children tend to be more flexible in new situations. They come across as calm and not easy to upset.

SAFETY *STAT!*

Short Answer

List the "7 rights for safe medication administration":

1. _____

2. _____

3. _____

4. _____

5. _____

6. _____

7. _____

DRUG FACTS

Short Answer Question

Certain medications should always be double-checked by two nurses. Institutional policy and procedures will guide the pediatric health-care team in how to best administer medications safely to a child; some may require that an RN be present as part of the safety check. Always know your health-care institution's policies about double-checking medications. Name six examples of high-alert medications that should have two nurses double-check them for safety.

1. _____

2. _____

3. _____

4. _____

5. _____

6. _____

TABLE COMPLETION

Pediatric nurses rely on their knowledge of developmental theory to guide their interactions, expectations, and teaching. Theory provides a framework to make sense of childhood behaviors. Complete the table, naming the four significant theorists associated with each of the theoretical frameworks provided.

Theoretical Framework	Theorist
Psychosocial development	
Cognitive development	
Psychosexual development	
Moral development	

SAFETY *STAT!*

Concept Map

Complete the concept map (Fig. 20.1) with information related to the concept of "new morbidity" concerning children's educational experiences and school environments.

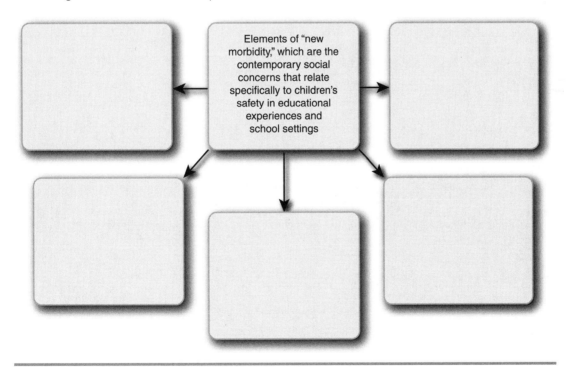

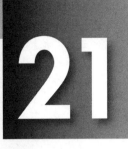

Health Promotion of the Infant: Birth to One Year

Name: _____

Date: _____

Course: _____

Instructor: _____

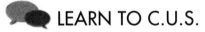 LEARN TO C.U.S.

Short Answer Questions

The pediatric nurse notices that his colleague is administering medications to an infant who has been hospitalized for cellulitis of the face and neck without double-checking the medication safe dose range for the infant's weight or the final dose concentration.

1. What is the protocol for safe medication administration for infants?

2. How would you respond to this nurse?

_____

_____

_____

TRUE OR FALSE QUESTIONS

1. _____ Infants need to develop a sense of trust in their environment and with their caregivers. This can be accomplished by allowing the infant to cry for their needs and learn delayed gratification.

2. _____ Infants experience both stranger anxiety and separation anxiety. These normal and expected behaviors begin to be displayed at 6 months of age.

3. _____ All infants generally follow a consistent pattern of growth and development with precise time frames expected for each milestone.

MATCHING EXERCISE

Match the correct definition with each vocabulary word.

_____ 1. Type of play infants are
            engaged with

_____ 2. 12 month infant screen-
            ing is done to detect
            this disorder

_____ 3. Age an infant can
            roll over

_____ 4. Common injury for an
            infant

A. 6 to 8 months

B. Retinopathy of prematurity

C. 3 to 4 months

D. Burns

E. Solitary

F. Iron deficiency anemia

G. Associative

H. Falls

CULTURAL CONSIDERATIONS

Short Answer Question

Infants should follow a sequence of solid food introduction. Although the introduction of food is influenced by a family's ethnic background or culture, the nurse should provide anticipatory guidance in infant food introduction in order to safely identify whether there is a food allergy. Describe, in order, what and when various groups of solid food should be introduced to the infant:

1. _____

2. _____

3. _____

4. _____

5. _____

6. _____

CASE STUDY

Short Answer Question

Ted, a new father of a full-term infant daughter, is planning on taking an online safety course for new parents. State 10 essential components of a first-time-parent safety course for bringing home a newborn.

1. _____

2. _____

3. _____

4. _____

5. _____

6. _____

7. _____

8. _____

9. _____

10. _____

CASE STUDY

Fill-in-the-Blank Question

Danielle, a 9-month-old infant, is a well-nourished older infant who displays expected language, motor, and psychosocial development for her age. She has no significant past medical history other than one ear infection and two typical colds. She was born full-term and her height and weight are within the 50th percentile on a Center of Disease Control (CDC) growth chart.

According to Erik Erikson's _____ theory, Danielle is in the

_____ versus _____ stage of infant development. The behaviors that Danielle's parents are most concerned about stem from her oral gratification developmental

stage that causes her to want to _____.

SAFETY *STAT!*

Short Answer Question

Thermoregulation is very important for a newborn infant. Describe two ways in which a nurse can provide support for newborn thermoregulation:

1. _____

2. _____

PATIENT TEACHING GUIDELINES

True or False Question

_____ In a dominant disorder, both sets of genes passed on to the infant come from both parents.

CONCEPTUAL CORNERSTONE
Fill-in-the-Blank Question

Family-centered care provides a foundation in which to interact with and support new

families. Components of family-centered care include _____,

_____, _____, and _____.

Health Promotion of the Toddler

22

Name: _____

Date: _____

Course: _____

Instructor: _____

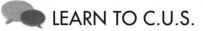 LEARN TO C.U.S.

Short Answer Question

A pediatric nurse notices that the mother of a child is willing to assist in the administration of her son's oral medication. She readily accepts the responsibilities but wants to do it on "her family's typical time." She takes the medications from the nurse and places the oral syringes into the drawer of the table next to the child's hospital bed. There are other hospitalized children in the room.

What are your appropriate responses to this mother about this safety concern?

_____

_____

_____

CONCEPTUAL CORNERSTONE: CULTURE

Short Answer Questions

Find a partner and write out the answers to the following items. Keep in mind cultural considerations.

1. Identify deviations from expected developmental milestones during the toddler period.

_____

_____

2. Select toddler-friendly and safe foods that represent a good source of nutrition.

_____

_____

3. Identify ways to maintain safe home environments for the active toddler and include essential components for parent teaching.

_____

_____

4. How would a pediatric nurse assess for a safe hospital environment for a hospitalized toddler, including identifying basic safety strategies.

_____

_____

5. Select an appropriate car seat for the toddler and describe how to place it in a car.

_____

_____

6. Select appropriate safe and challenging toys that encourage cognitive and motor development, including balance.

_____

_____

CONCEPTUAL CORNERSTONE: DEVELOPMENT
Fill-in-the-Blank Questions

1. According to Erickson's psychosocial developmental theory, a toddler will be struggling with a sense of _____ versus _____

2. "_____   _____ and _____" is a phrase used to describe the picky eating behaviors and food refusal behaviors found frequently in children who are in the toddler developmental period.

THERAPEUTIC COMMUNICATION

Matching Exercise

_____ 1. Negativism

_____ 2. Separation anxiety

_____ 3. Autonomy

_____ 4. Stranger anxiety

_____ 5. Parallel play

A. Anxiety experienced by an older infant or young child when separated by their primary caregiver(s)

B. Anxiety experienced by an older infant or young child when they encounter a new person(s) in their environment

C. Behavior of a young child marked by resistance or retreat; often associated with tantruming

D. The actual or desired state of independence; may be considered a state of separation of the child's primary caregiver

E. A form of play associated with the toddler developmental stage in which the child does not play with another toddler, but plays close by, often back to back, with separate toys that they do not have to share

THERAPEUTIC COMMUNICATION

Review Question

Talking with toddlers can be a challenge. Due to their developmental stage of autonomy versus sham and doubt, they often respond to requests with saying, "No!"

Which of the following strategies to engage a toddler in procedures, such as immunizations, medication administration, or wound care would be appropriate? (*select all that apply*)

1. Offer two choices to the child.
2. Immediately request the assistance of at least two other health-care professionals.
3. Use medical play and anatomically correct dolls.
4. Tell the young child the medication is "yummy" and tastes like candy.
5. Solicit the help of the parents or guardian.
6. Use distraction.
7. Ask the parent to leave so the nurse can take charge of the situation.
8. Begin by explaining the details of the procedure to the child.
9. Reward the child's cooperation by saying they will receive a sticker or a prize for cooperating.

SAFETY *STAT!*

Review Question

Which of the following statements represents the need to provide more safety teaching to the parents of a toddler being seen in the clinic?

1. We always provide supervision when our child is playing outside, in the park, or by the pool.
2. We use a car seat each and every time we drive without exception.
3. We have our hot water heater turned to 115°F.
4. We have our cleaning supplies and antifreeze stored in a closet in the garage where our child does not play.

PATIENT TEACHING GUIDELINES

True or False Questions

1. _____ After age 1 year, low-fat milk (2%) can be offered to a toddler.

2. _____ Food lags, or picky eating, has been strongly associated with weight loss.

3. _____ Bedtime rituals are no longer important to an older toddler as they have mastered their bedtime sleeping time and place.

4. _____ The most appropriate response to a toddler stating there is a monster in their closet is to say that even though the parent does not see the monster, they will leave the bedroom door open and the night light on.

PATIENT TEACHING GUIDELINES

Short Answer Questions

1. The annual weight gain of a toddler is how many kilograms per year on average?

   _____

2. How many inches will a toddler's head circumference grow between 1 and 2 years of age?

   _____

3. How would one describe the walking stance of a toddler?

   _____

Health Promotion of the Preschooler

23

Name: _____

Date: _____

Course: _____

Instructor: _____

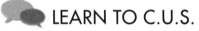 LEARN TO C.U.S.

Short Answer Question

The pediatric nurse working in homecare for children with chronic health conditions or disabilities is visiting a family whose child is experiencing mild respiratory distress, low-grade fevers, and fatigue. The child has a history of cystic fibrosis, which has required several inpatient stays in the last few years. Upon assessment, the nurse finds the child with clinical signs of dehydration, increased work of breathing, and an oral temperature of 100.8°F. The mother states that she can manage the child at home and plans on continuing the antibiotics prescribed for the child during the last clinic visit 6 days ago. What concerns do you have for this situation? How might you address your concerns with the mother?

_____

_____

CONCEPTUAL CORNERSTONE: DEVELOPMENT

True or False Questions

1. _____ Preschool children cannot understand the concept of time even when references are made about the present, past, and future.

2. _____ Preschool children's vocabulary should be at least 500 words by the time the child is 5 years old.

3. _____ Preschool children often display mistaken perceptions of reality. This phenomenon is called magical thinking.

MATCHING EXERCISES

Match the correct definition with each vocabulary word.

_____ 1. Type of play preschool children engage in

_____ 2. Preschool vision screening is done to detect

_____ 3. One cause for feelings of guilt

_____ 4. Common injury for preschooler

A. Magical thinking

B. Drowning

C. Sibling rivalry

D. Parallel play

E. Myopia and amblyopia

F. Associative play

G. Playground falls

H. Tricycle accidents

TEAM WORKS

Short Answer Questions

Parents have brought in a preschool child into the public health clinic for a tuberculosis (TB) test that has been recommended by their private preschool homecare provider. The child has had a potential exposure to an adult with active TB. The parents, upon assessment of the child's past medical history, state that she has never had any childhood immunizations beyond the first hepatitis B vaccine after birth. They state they do not "believe in or support" administering immunizations to their children. Note the four childhood immunizations that are due during this child's preschool period:

1. _____

2. _____

3. _____

4. _____

TEAM WORKS

Short Answer Questions

The pediatric nurse notifies all members of the health-care team about the parents' refusal of immunizations for the child. The team assembles briefly and decides to educate the parents on why childhood immunizations are important. List three items for discussion with the parents:

1. _____

2. _____

3. _____

REVIEW QUESTION

A 3½-year-old boy is hospitalized for a fractured humerus obtained when he fell off of a snow mobile while his uncle was driving. What could the nurse do to foster his developmental milestone of a sense of initiative?

1. Allow the child to play video games with another child his own age.

2. Provide the child with books to read with his sibling when his family visits each night.

3. Allow the child to administer his own oral medications from an oral syringe.

4. Provide the child an opportunity to view a developmentally appropriate video about what to expect when a child is hospitalized.

CASE STUDY

Short Answer Question

Christina is a 3-year-old girl who is demonstrating normal and expected motor milestones for her developmental stage. She is healthy and active. List five motor accomplishments you would expect her to demonstrate during play:

1. _____

2. _____

3. _____

4. _____

5. _____

CULTURAL CONSIDERATIONS

Fill-in-the-Blank Questions

Christina, a 3-year-old Russian girl, has been attending preschool 5 days a week for greater than 8 hours per day. Both of her parents work full time away from the home and require a short commute in opposite directions. She has one older sibling, Logan, who attends kindergarten followed by a school-based aftercare program. Her parents have expressed concern to the preschool administrator that because her mother announced that she was going to have a baby, Christina's behavior in the evenings has been progressively more toddler-like with enuresis nightly, tantrums, food refusal, and aggression toward the family pet. Over the course of the last week, Christina has been getting out of bed during the night seeking her parents' comfort for concerns that there is a "monster" under her bed. The parents do not allow her to come into their bed, because their cultural practice is to promote independence. In order to help this family, knowledge of her developmental stage is needed.

According to Erik Erikson's _____ theory, Christina is in the

_____ versus _____ stage of development. The

behaviors that Christina's parents are concerned about stem from her _____
thought processes that occur during the preschool period. To help the child cope with a new baby, the parents should reassure Christina that she is loved and will always be important to her parents and can help them with the new baby when he/she arrives.

REVIEW QUESTION

As the pediatric nurse is preparing to take vital signs on a preschool child in for a well-child checkup in the clinic, the child bursts out crying and says the cuff and tubing are going to turn into a monster and "cut her arm off." The nurse realizes this is an example of which type of thinking?

1. Magical thinking

2. Associative thinking

3. Egocentrism

4. Animism

Health Promotion of the School-Aged Child

24

Name: _____

Date: _____

Course: _____

Instructor: _____

PATIENT TEACHING GUIDELINES
Fill-in-the-Blank Questions

1. The term used to describe the set of "baby teeth" that shed during the school-age developmental period are called _____ _____.

2. According to Erickson's Theory, school-age children are struggling with a sense of _____ versus _____.

3. During the later years of the school-age developmental stage, the demonstration of the beginning of sexual maturity of a young girl is called _____.

CONCEPTUAL CORNERSTONE: GROWTH AND DEVELOPMENT
Matching Exercise

_____ 1. Freud's psycho-
sexual state for
the school-age
child

_____ 2. A common type
of injury during
the school-age
period

_____ 3. The age at which
puberty normally
begins in girls

_____ 4. The age at which
precocious pu-
berty may begin
as young as

_____ 5. The stages in
which play in the
early school-age
period moves
from and to

_____ 6. The term by
which tempera-
ment can also be
referred to

A. 8 to 12 years of age

B. Before 8 years of age

C. Latency

D. Over-use syndrome

E. Reactivity

F. Informal; from free to structured with rules

CONCEPTUAL CORNERSTONE
Fill-in-the-Blank Questions

1. Comfort
Providing comfort and pain control is an important role for the pediatric nurse caring for a

school-age child. Children at this developmental level can use _____
pain tools and should be encouraged to describe their pain, state the location, and respond to a

_____ pain-scale tool.

2. Development
During middle childhood, the average weight gain for boys and girls is between

_____ and _____ pounds per year, and

the average height increase is _____ inches per year.

TEAM WORKS: HEALTH, WELLNESS, AND ILLNESS

Short Answer Questions

1. You have been asked to participate in the development and implementation of a wellness fair for a large local middle school (6th to 8th graders) in your community. You have recruited nursing students from the local community college to assist you by setting up and staffing several interactive booths to engage the school-age children in activities that would interest them. List five topics for booths at this wellness fair:

   1. _____

   2. _____

   3. _____

   4. _____

   5. _____

2. Precocious puberty can occur during the school-age period. List three factors that place a school-age child at risk for the development of precocious puberty:

   1. _____

   2. _____

   3. _____

3. Children in the school-age period are very prone to injuries because their muscles are still growing and are not as functionally mature as they will be once they reach adolescence. State two reasons that school-age children are prone to injuries:

   1. _____

   2. _____

LEARN TO C.U.S.

Short Answer Question

A pediatric nurse is employed as a district school nurse for a large urban school district. An elementary school secretary calls to inform the school nurse that an 8-year-old second-grade child fell from the top of a climbing structure onto the outdoor mats on the playground. The secretary said she had already notified the parents and the father was leaving work to come and pick up the child. She said there were conflicting stories from the other children and playground supervisors about whether or not the child lost consciousness briefly. The secretary told the nurse she was just informing him or her, in case paperwork needs to be filed. How should the school nurse respond, using the Learn to C.U.S. method of communication?

_____

_____

_____

_____

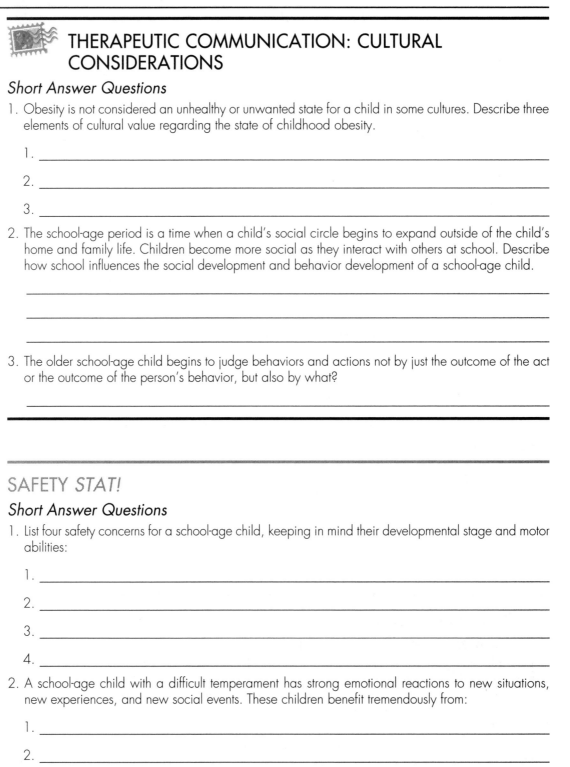

THERAPEUTIC COMMUNICATION: CULTURAL CONSIDERATIONS

Short Answer Questions

1. Obesity is not considered an unhealthy or unwanted state for a child in some cultures. Describe three elements of cultural value regarding the state of childhood obesity.

    1. _____

    2. _____

    3. _____

2. The school-age period is a time when a child's social circle begins to expand outside of the child's home and family life. Children become more social as they interact with others at school. Describe how school influences the social development and behavior development of a school-age child.

    _____

    _____

    _____

3. The older school-age child begins to judge behaviors and actions not by just the outcome of the act or the outcome of the person's behavior, but also by what?

    _____

SAFETY *STAT!*

Short Answer Questions

1. List four safety concerns for a school-age child, keeping in mind their developmental stage and motor abilities:

    1. _____

    2. _____

    3. _____

    4. _____

2. A school-age child with a difficult temperament has strong emotional reactions to new situations, new experiences, and new social events. These children benefit tremendously from:

    1. _____

    2. _____

PATIENT TEACHING GUIDELINES
Review Questions

1. The pediatric nurse has been asked to present information to school-age children in a 5th grade class concerning nutrition and healthy eating. While deciding how to best prepare a lesson plan, the nurse considers appropriate material. Which of the following would not be included in the lesson plan?
   1. A list of the major food groups with several food examples for each group
   2. An introduction to appropriate serving sizes
   3. A lesson on food labels to learn required information on fats, carbohydrates, and calories
   4. A discussion on the importance of dieting

2. School-age children enjoy time with family. In order to promote healthy family dynamics, school-age children express an appreciation for which the following?
   1. Spending time alone with each parent
   2. Having all members of the family interact together
   3. Having private sibling time for bonding
   4. Showing appreciation for parents by supporting their time alone

3. School-age children demonstrate their ability to understand the social environment around them. This includes understanding their parents' roles by:
   1. Understanding the role of each gender
   2. Understanding the role of a working parent
   3. Understanding the divergent role of each parent in the home
   4. Understanding the role of their teacher in society

4. Play continues to be an important aspect of the older school-age child. Which of the following describes the type of play of this developmental stage?
   1. Cooperation and teamwork
   2. Associative
   3. Playing team sports with same-sex teams
   4. Negotiative

5. Play during the school-age period enhances the development of a sense of:
   1. Self-identify as the child learns who they are in the world
   2. Autonomy as the child learns to occupy and entertain themselves
   3. Morality as the child conforms to social norms
   4. Industry as the child completes puzzles and homework

PATIENT TEACHING GUIDELINES
True or False Questions

1. _____ The school-age period, which spans the longest of the developmental stages, is also known as the *latency* period.

2. _____ The school-age developmental stage, according to Erikson, is defined by the sense of industry.

3. _____ Children within the school-age developmental period participate in an associative type of play, which is marked by engagement of play activities that are same-sex partnerships.

SAFETY *STAT!*

True or False Questions

1. _____ Because hearing screening is very important during the school-age developmental period, the American Speech and Hearing Association recommends that an audiologist train screeners.

2. _____ Hearing screening is usually tested in the school-age period by testing several tones presented at varying levels of pitch. Rescreening should be done with at least a 1-week interval if the child fails the first time.

3. _____ Besides failing a hearing screening test, children with a bad odor or discharge/drainage from their ears should have their hearing checked as soon as possible.

PATIENT TEACHING GUIDELINES

Complete the following concept map (Fig. 24.1) with teaching points to a parent of a school-age child who is concerned about her child's third lice infestation.

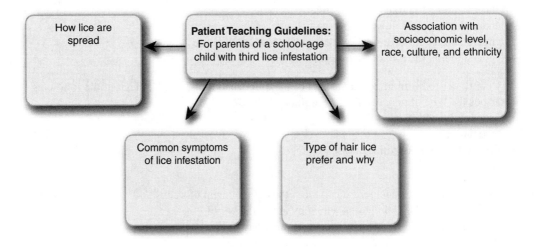

Health Promotion of the Adolescent

25

Name: _____

Date: _____

Course: _____

Instructor: _____

CONCEPTUAL CORNERSTONE: DEVELOPMENT

True or False Questions

1. _____ Adolescence is a time of maturing in the area of moral development and spirituality. Teens begin questioning existing moral values, yet according to Kohlberg's theory, the adolescent is not yet able to critically evaluate a moral dilemma and is not yet able to discern aspects about his or her own set of morals.

2. _____ According to Kohlberg's theory, the stage of moral development for a teen is called the *preconventional level of morality.*

PATIENT TEACHING GUIDELINES

Short Answer Question

A nurse caring for a teen should explain expected changes to the child and their family. List five physical or physiological changes that can be expected during the rapid growth and development of adolescents:

1. _____

2. _____

3. _____

4. _____

5. _____

CONCEPTUAL CORNERSTONE: DEVELOPMENT

Fill-in-the-Blank Question

Piaget, the well-known and widely accepted author of a _____

_____ _____, created four levels of cognitive development. According to Piaget's theory, adolescents are in the _____

_____ cognitive stage, which is marked by three distinct aspects:

(1) _____ _____,

(2) _____ _____, and

(3) _____ _____ _____.

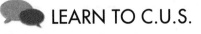 LEARN TO C.U.S.

Short Answer Question

A pediatric nurse is working in an adolescent health clinic. He overhears a teenager tell a story in the waiting room to another teen whom he had just met. The teens were discussing a new drug that was becoming popular in the high school's athletic team circles. The boys were making light conversation about how easy it is to get drugs at their schools. Although they did not disclose whether or not they had ever taken drugs or describe any current substance use, the nurse became concerned by the lightheartedness of the conversation. When each teen was brought in to an exam room for their appointments, the nurse decided to discuss with each teen his concerns about the prevalence of teen drug use. How might the nurse express his concerns using the Learn to C.U.S. model of communication?

C: _____

U: _____

S: _____

SAFETY *STAT!*

Table Completion: Normal Vital Signs for Adolescents

Temperature	
Heart Rate	
Blood Pressure	
Respiratory Rate	

CULTURAL CONSIDERATIONS

Short Answer Question

A middle-school teenage girl came into the adolescent health clinic for an immunization booster for tetanus and pertussis. She came wearing a headscarf that represents a cultural practice of covering her hair and head at all times while in public. While alone with her in the room, she became tearful and said she had been bullied earlier in the day by a group of girls who teased her about her scarf, telling her to remove it and stating that "she was either bald under there or had a head full of lice." Considering her cultural background, how might the pediatric nurse respond?

_____

_____

_____

_____

THERAPEUTIC COMMUNICATION

Short Answer Question

Suggest eight ways for improving communication between adults and teens.

1. _____

2. _____

3. _____

4. _____

5. _____

6. _____

7. _____

8. _____

SAFETY *STAT!*

True or False Question

_____ The best way to prevent cyberbullying during the early teenage years is to limit access to computers and have parents know all login and password information, including social media sites.

THERAPEUTIC COMMUNICATION

Short Answer Question

Sometimes when a teenager is admitted to the pediatric floor for a period of time of hospitalization, the pediatric nursing team can be challenged to establish a positive and trustworthy rapport. The teenager may see the nurse as an authoritative figure and may limit his or her discussion or disclosures with the nurse. If this is the case, the nurse may be challenged to develop a personal relationship that will assist in the recovery of the teen's health issue. List several ideas for activities that the nurse can use to engage the teen to promote communication, trust, and rapport.

_____

_____

_____

_____

_____

_____

_____

_____

_____

_____

_____

PATIENT TEACHING GUIDELINES

True or False Question

_____ Promoting healthy eating habits is important during the teen years. Consuming adequate calcium is often a challenge, especially for teenage girls. The recommended daily dose of elemental calcium for a teenager is no less than 1600 mg/day.

PATIENT TEACHING GUIDELINES

Table Completion

As teenagers grow, they experience physiological changes related to development. Complete the table with examples of each of the listed body changes.

Hormones are known to affect an adolescent's physical changes	
Genitals change as the teen matures	
Frontal lobe nerves become myelinated	

CONCEPTUAL CORNERSTONE: DEVELOPMENT

CONCEPT MAP COMPLETION

Complete the concept map with information you have learned about Freud's theory about psychosocial development (Fig. 25.1).

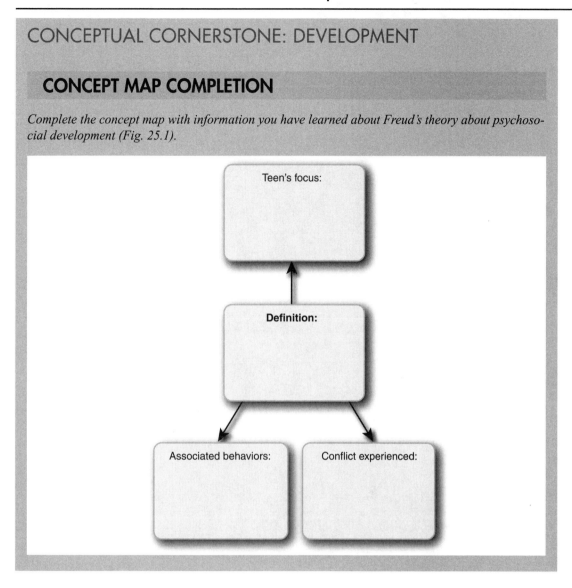

Pediatric Concerns and Considerations

The Hospitalized Child

26

Name: _____

Date: _____

Course: _____

Instructor: _____

💬 LEARN TO C.U.S.

Short Answer Questions

While receiving a report from a nurse, you are told that a young toddler has been left alone while his parents attended to issues at work. The plan, as described to you, is that the child will be alone for about 4 hours, and then a grandparent will come and stay with the child until one of the parents can return. The child has been admitted for a viral illness that causes respiratory distress and a history of recent severe reactive airway disease. You are told that the toddler is currently in a hospital bed with a nasal cannula with oxygen at 0.5 L/min. His IV is saline locked and he is not due for a respiratory treatment for 2 more hours.

1. What concerns do you have about this child?

   _____

   _____

   _____

   _____

   _____

2. Using the C.U.S. method of communication, how might you phrase your concerns to the off-going nurse?

   C: _____

   U: _____

   S: _____

THERAPEUTIC COMMUNICATION

True or False Questions

1. _____ Giving difficult news to parents about their preschool-age child's acute condition is best done at the bedside, where the parents can see the child and understand the condition.

2. _____ Family-centered care provides guidelines for implementing best practices for conferences in which a child's condition will be discussed and a treatment plan outlined. Parents should be included in the conference only after the plan of medical care is set and all team members have been informed.

3. _____ Older siblings should not be included in bedside rounds in which a child's condition is discussed as it might frighten them.

TEAM WORKS: COMMUNICATING UP THE CHAIN OF COMMAND

Short Answer Question

You are caring for a young child hospitalized after a surgical procedure to lyse adhesions from a previous severe ruptured appendectomy that caused scarring. While providing care, the nurse notes that the recently postoperative child is more tachycardic than the previous baseline, is pale, and is complaining of pain rated an 8 on a Wong-Baker FACES® Pain Rating Scale. What is the reporting sequence that would be the safest for the child? Give a rationale for your answer.

_____

_____

_____

_____

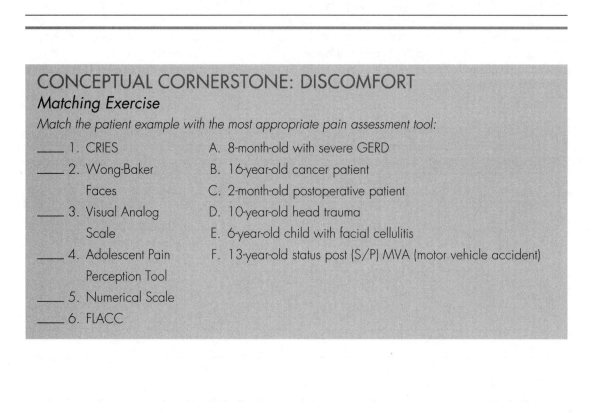

CONCEPTUAL CORNERSTONE: DISCOMFORT

Matching Exercise

Match the patient example with the most appropriate pain assessment tool:

_____ 1. CRIES

_____ 2. Wong-Baker Faces

_____ 3. Visual Analog Scale

_____ 4. Adolescent Pain Perception Tool

_____ 5. Numerical Scale

_____ 6. FLACC

A. 8-month-old with severe GERD

B. 16-year-old cancer patient

C. 2-month-old postoperative patient

D. 10-year-old head trauma

E. 6-year-old child with facial cellulitis

F. 13-year-old status post (S/P) MVA (motor vehicle accident)

CULTURAL CONSIDERATIONS: PERCEPTIONS ABOUT PAIN MANAGEMENT

Short Answer Question

Including a family's culture is an important part of pain management. A tool was developed by Baker and Wong (1987) to consider all aspects of a child's pain experience that includes the input of the parents. Define the QUESTT pain assessment mnemonic and give an example of each component for a 5-year-old Muslim girl whose parents express concern about the administration of postoperative narcotics.

Q: _____

U: _____

E: _____

S: _____

T: _____

T: _____

PATIENT TEACHING GUIDELINES

Short Answer Questions

1. List five emotional reactions a sibling might express while a younger family member is hospitalized for a recent diagnosis of neuroblastoma that requires a lengthy hospitalization.

   1. _____

   2. _____

   3. _____

   4. _____

   5. _____

2. State why it is important to discuss and acknowledge these common emotional reactions with the parents or caregiver.

   _____

   _____

   _____

3. Parents who are concerned about their hospitalized child experiencing pain question the nurse about the side effects of multiple doses of narcotics for pain control. After explaining the need to control the child's acute pain, the nurse presents the parents with examples of the consequences of untreated pain. List seven examples of these consequences:

1. _____

2. _____

3. _____

4. _____

5. _____

6. _____

7. _____

CONCEPTUAL CORNERSTONE: DISCOMFORT

Draw an Illustration

Draw an illustration of the following three pain scales used in children:
Wong-Baker FACES Pain Rating Scale:

FLACC Scale:

Numeric Scale:

SAFETY *STAT!*: MEDICATION ADMINISTRATION AT HOME

True or False Questions

1. _____ In situations in which extra doses of medication have been taken at home (for instance, pain medications that are not used), the hospital protocols are for families to dispose of the medications by crushing them and putting them down the sink, or by flushing them in the toilet. This procedure is set up for safety to prevent accidental poisoning, with the remaining quantity of the drug staying in the home.

2. _____ Topical medications are frequently ordered for a variety of reasons in pediatric health care. It is important to teach the family that, in general, topical medications should be applied generously in order for the medication to be effective.

SAFETY *STAT!*

Table Completion

Complete the table below with a description of how to collect each specimen from a child.

Specimen Collected	Description of Collecting the Specimen
Clean Catch: Undiapered Child	
Clean Catch: Diapered Child	
Sterile Catheterization	
24-Hour Urine Collection	
Stool Specimens	
Sputum Specimens	
RSV Specimens	
MRSE Specimens	
Influenza A and B Specimen Collection	
Phlebotomy	

TEAM WORKS

Short Answer Question

Define the term *compliance* as it relates to post-hospitalization medication regimens. Give a hypothetical example of a situation in which compliance is an issue.

_____

_____

_____

SAFETY *STAT!*

Fill-in-the-Blank Question

Parents of children of all ages often feel _____ when outside work or family responsibilities pull them from the hospitalized child's bedside. The parents must hear from the nurse

that the child will be kept _____, _____ and

_____ _____ for in their absence.

Acutely Ill Children and Their Needs

27

Name: _____

Date: _____

Course: _____

Instructor: _____

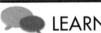 LEARN TO C.U.S.

Short Answer Question

You are caring for a young infant who is hospitalized for a rule-out bacterial urinary tract infection. Although blood and urine cultures are pending, the child is currently being treated with a broad-spectrum antibiotic until sensitivities can be determined to match the microbial culprit with the correct antibiotic. At the beginning of your shift, the child is demonstrating tachycardia, tachypnea, and lethargy. After reporting the findings to the charge nurse, you prepare to discuss the child with the rounding physician. How might you organize your concerns?

C: _____

U: _____

S: _____

TEAM WORKS

Short Answer Question

Who are the nine members of a rapid response/code blue team and what is each of their roles?

1. _____

2. _____

3. _____

4. _____

5. _____

6. _____

7. _____

8. _____

9. _____

THERAPEUTIC COMMUNICATION

Short Answer Question

Describe how you would phrase the question to parents about whether or not the family might want to stay present during a rapid response by a modified pediatric code blue team for a child having a severe allergic response to the administration of intravenous medication.

_____

_____

_____

_____

_____

SAFETY *STAT!*

True or False Questions

1. _____ Basic emergency equipment found on a pediatric crash cart would include the following: color-coded length-based resuscitation tape, oxygen, airway supplies, IV supplies, laboratory supplies, backboard, suction equipment, monitor, and oxygen tank.

2. _____ Research has shown that most families would like to be present for at least part of the attempted resuscitative process.

3. _____ The mnemonic AVPU stands for a quick mental status exam that covers: awake, responds to voice, responds to painful stimuli, and unresponsive to painful stimuli.

SAFETY *STAT!*

Review Questions

1. Which of the following medications would the pediatric health-care team staff want to have available for an emergency response in health-care settings where childhood immunizations are administered? (*select all that apply*)
   1. Ranitidine oral solution
   2. Diphenhydramine injection
   3. Diphenhydramine oral solution
   4. Epinephrine 1:1,000 injection
   5. Methylprednisolone injection
2. Epiglottitis is a life-threatening infection and inflammation of the epiglottis. The most important aspect of responding to an emergency associated with airway obstruction from this infection is to:
   1. Prepare for a complete cardiopulmonary arrest.
   2. Prepare the child for rapid surgery.
   3. Administer an antibiotic as ordered.
   4. Obtain a throat culture but use a tongue blade and cotton swab.

NURSING CARE PLAN: Short Answer Question

Write a nursing diagnosis and a corresponding nursing goal (patient-oriented) for the family of a young infant who has been admitted to the pediatric unit after having an acute life-threatening event.

Nursing diagnosis: _____

Nursing (patient-oriented) goal: _____

PATIENT TEACHING GUIDELINES

Short Answer Question

A child is being discharged with a prescription for an Epi-Pen® for a longstanding medical history of highly reactive severe asthma. The father asks about the need for the pen to be available to the child at all times. How would the nurse describe to the father some tips on how to maintain access to the life-saving Epi-Pen®?

_____

_____

_____

_____

SAFETY *STAT!*

Short Answer Question

The nursing staff of an emergency room is responding to a child who presents in acute dehydration from having emesis and diarrhea for the last 3 days. The child is estimated to have lost at least 10% of his previous weight. A series of three boluses have been ordered to resuscitate the child's fluid status. Describe the solution that will be used for the intravenous administration and calculate the fluid bolus if the child weighs 27 pounds.

Solution _____

Weight in kilograms _____

Calculated bolus quantity _____

SAFETY *STAT!*

Matching Exercise

_____ 1. Broselow® tape

_____ 2. Rapid response team

_____ 3. Code blue

_____ 4. Shock

A. A phrase used to describe an actual or pending cardiopulmonary arrest

B. A clinical syndrome marked by inadequate oxygenation and perfusion of tissues and organs at the cellular level due to markedly low systemic blood pressure

C. A color-coded length-based resuscitative tape system for emergency response based on a child's actual or estimated weight

D. A designated team response designed to rapidly assemble at a child's bedside or clinic room to provide emergency response skills and resuscitation if needed

SAFETY *STAT!*

Short Answer Question

Describe how an intraosseous needle is used in pediatrics.

SAFETY *STAT!*

Acutely Ill Children: Labeling Tracheostomy Equipment

Label the parts of a tracheostomy tube (Fig. 27.1).

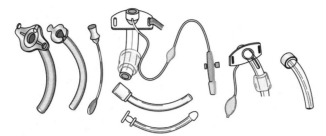

SAFETY *STAT!*

Complete the Concept Map

The pediatric health-care team is going to transfer a child from a small acute care pediatric unit in a rural hospital to the pediatric intensive care unit (PICU) in a city 25 miles away. Fill out the safety concept map (Fig. 27.2) based on the required preparation for the child to be transferred.

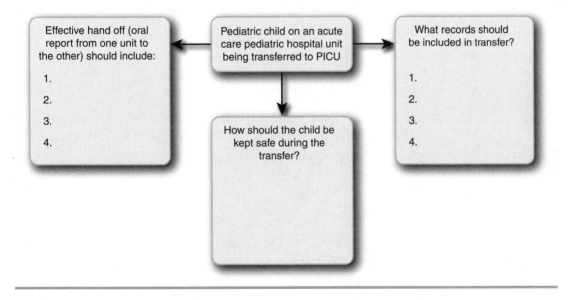

The Abused Child

28

Name: _____

Date: _____

Course: _____

Instructor: _____

💬 LEARN TO C.U.S.

Short Answer Question

You are a newly graduated nurse who is working in a busy pediatric outpatient clinic where 50 to 60 children are seen on a daily basis. You are performing vital signs and an initial intake assessment on an adolescent mother who is bringing her 3-month-old infant for her first set of immunizations after the child had received the first hepatitis vaccine after birth. You weigh the infant, measure length and head circumference, and plot your findings on a national growth chart. You become alarmed that the infant is demonstrating a third percentile for each of the three measurements. You become concerned. You orient the family to the room and tell them you will be back to provide care.

1. What are your next steps and whom do you contact?
2. How can you phrase your concerns using the Learn to C.U.S. method of communication?

C: _____

U: _____

S: _____

TEAM WORKS

Short Answer Question

You have been requested by a local school district to conduct an annual development conference of teachers and school administrators for a public preschool on several topics related to young children's health. One topic requested is an update on the most important topics related to identifying signs of child neglect and abuse. What are the top 10 major categories you will want to cover in your presentation? Write an outline of topics you will cover:

1. _____

2. _____

3. _____

4. _____

5. _____

6. _____

7. _____

8. _____

9. _____

10. _____

CONCEPTUAL CORNERSTONES: GROWTH AND DEVELOPMENT

Short Answer Question

A family comes into the pediatric emergency department with a young child suffering from severe respiratory distress and high fever. The child is 3 years old but appears to be very small and thin for the stated age. The family has two other children and is accompanied by an older gentleman in a wheelchair. The family states they just recently immigrated to the United States and the family currently has no source of income. They are staying in a small room of an apartment of a cousin. The other children are ages 5 and 7. The family has no insurance and expressed grave concern about finances and their ability to pay for any prescriptions or copayments that may be required to secure care for their ill child.

The child is demonstrating a fever of 102.3°F. The child is tachypnic at 44 breaths per minute. The child has mild poor skin turgor and has not voided in many hours. There is a history of asthma in the family but this child has no history of reactive airway disease and no previous experiences of respiratory distress. Upon further assessment, the child is demonstrating delays in expected motor and verbal development. The pediatric team is concerned about the possibility of this child being neglected and wants to determine whether the neglect is intentional or unintentional. Describe what your next steps would be in this complicated clinical scenario:

_____

_____

_____

_____

_____

THERAPEUTIC COMMUNICATION

Short Answer Questions

A young infant has been hospitalized for severe malnutrition and delays in expected growth and development. During the hospitalization, the single mother of the child has not visited. The maternal grandmother is at the bedside throughout each evening and stays many hours with the infant, holding her and caring for her. The grandmother describes how the mother is "taking drugs," is "out every night," and has no employment. When the infant turned 1 month of age, the mother and child moved in with the grandmother as they faced homelessness in their previous living circumstances. While assessing the child at the beginning of the shift, the grandmother bursts out crying and asks for help in the situation.

1. How would you respond to the grandmother?
   Immediate response:

   _____

   _____

2. What resources and referrals can you make to assist the family?
   Resources and referrals:

   _____

   _____

   _____

PATIENT TEACHING GUIDELINES

Short Answer Question

A single father comes into the outpatient pediatric clinic with three children under the age of 5. He states that he is currently unemployed and is responsible for the children during the day when his wife is working. He is forthcoming in saying that his patience is tried many times a day and he wants to know some ideas for calmly disciplining his children. There is no evidence of abuse noted but the children have dirty clothes and their personal hygiene is poor. Give three ideas for the father to use positive parenting discipline for his children all under the age of 5.

1. _____
2. _____
3. _____

TEAM WORKS

Fill-in-the-Blank Question

In general, there are four categories of mandatory child abuse reporters. These four categories include

all _____ _____ _____,

_____ _____ _____,

_____ _____ _____, and all

_____ _____ _____

_____.

True or False Question

_____ Munchausen syndrome by proxy (MSBP) is a title for harm or significant injury to a child by another individual, often the father, who typically has some health-care knowledge and who inflicts harm to child in order to receive attention from others.

NURSING DIAGNOSIS
Short Answer Question

Write a nursing diagnosis for a young child who has experienced Munchausen syndrome by proxy:

_____

LABS & DIAGNOSTICS
Short Answer Question

When caring for a child who has experienced intentional injuries and is a suspected victim of child abuse, a variety of laboratory evaluations may be ordered. Name six possible tests that are used to evaluate evidence of child abuse.

1. _____

2. _____

3. _____

4. _____

5. _____

6. _____

Table Completion

Fill in the table based on the information and care needed for a child who has been abused.

Common behavioral signs of abuse in childhood:	
Maintaining safety for the child includes at least the following three areas:	
Possible physical indicators of abuse (list three):	
A rare form of child abuse where the mother has a mental health disorder and causes the child to have multiple tests and treatments:	

SAFETY STAT!

CONCEPT MAP COMPLETION

It is the responsibility of the pediatric health-care team to keep an abused child safe from further harm or injury. Complete the concept map (Fig. 28.1) of the following steps that the health-care team should use in the care and protection of a child who has been a victim of child abuse.

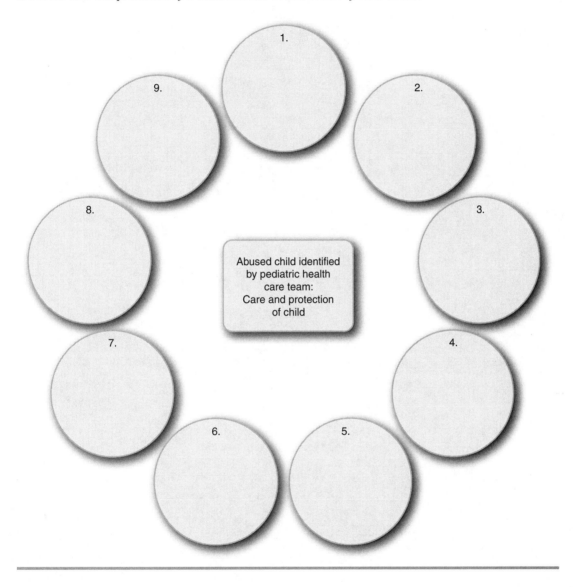

unit EIGHT

Deviations in Pediatric Health

Child With a Neurological Condition

29

Name: _____

Date: _____

Course: _____

Instructor: _____

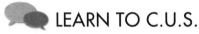 **LEARN TO C.U.S.**

Short Answer Question

A physician has written an order for a 13-year-old child with severe encephalopathy to receive Lorazepam 2 mg/kg STAT for seizure activity not controlled by her daily anticonvulsant therapy. As you diligently look up the safe dosage range for this child who weighs only 88 pounds, you see that the ordered dose of medication far exceeds the recommended maximum dose for her age, weight, and diagnosis. Using the Learn to C.U.S method of communication, how might you convey your concerns to the primary care provider who wrote the order?

C: _____

U: _____

S: _____

THERAPEUTIC COMMUNICATION

Short Answer Question

A grieving grandfather is at the bedside of a teenage boy who suffered a severe head concussion while playing football. The teen's admitting diagnosis was a subdural hematoma, concussion, and traumatic brain injury. The teen is currently asleep as the grandfather visits his bedside. How might you provide emotional support to this grandfather who was at the football game when the child suffered the accident?

_____

_____

_____

CULTURAL CONSIDERATIONS

Short Answer Question

An 8-year-old child with a near drowning diagnosis has been transferred to your rehabilitation unit for care. He is nonresponsive, has fixed and dilated pupils, is experiencing seizure activity frequently, and is a being treated for severe four-lobe pneumonia associated with the near-drowning episode. The parents' religious beliefs value life above all else and want everything done for this child. He is currently NPO due to his state of coma and is at a high risk of aspiration. They approach you at the nursing station with a thermos of homemade broth asking if you can assist them with trying to feed the child. What would you do next? What are your safety concerns?

_____

_____

_____

SAFETY *STAT!*

Labeling Exercise

Identify the following in Figure 29.1 of a ventricular-peritoneal shunt in a young child: the site of entry into the ventricle, the valve, the extra tubing, and where the tubing lies under the skin.

Ventriculoperitoneal (VP) Shunt

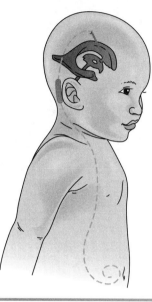

TEAM WORKS

True or False Questions

1. _____ The highest priority for a team responding to a child presenting with a head injury is to prepare the child for a high-level diagnostic imaging, such as an MRI or a CT scan.

2. _____ The pediatric health-care team must ensure that a child who is experiencing a full grand mal seizure with tonic-clonic movements is safe. The best way to ensure safety during a seizure is to hold the child carefully down on the floor to minimize any trauma that could occur.

CONCEPTUAL CORNERSTONE

Review Questions

1. Sensory perception is a concept associated with pediatric neurologic disorders. How is this concept defined?
   1. Sensory perception pertains to the intact state of the child's 12 cranial nerves.
   2. Sensory perception relates to the child's ability to experience and process sensory information.
   3. Sensory perception relates directly to pain and the perception of discomfort.
   4. Sensory perception relates to all neurologic structures that take in and process information.
2. A family presents to the pediatric clinic stating that their child is not responding to naturopathic herbs administered for the child's severe headache. While caring for this child with confirmed migraine headaches, the pediatric health-care team knows that which type of headache is associated with nausea, vomiting, and sensitivity to sound and light?
   1. Cluster headache
   2. Chronic daily headache
   3. Tension headache
   4. Migraine headache

TEAM WORKS

Short Answer Question

You have been requested to gather supplies to assist the charge nurse in assessing a child's cranial nerves I, III, and XI. First, name each cranial nerve. Then note the function of each nerve and the supplies you would gather to test each nerve's functioning.

Cranial nerve I:

Name: _____

Function: _____

Supplies for testing: _____

Cranial nerve III:

Name: _____

Function: _____

Supplies for testing: _____

Cranial nerve XI:

Name: _____

Function: _____

Supplies for testing: _____

LABS & DIAGNOSTICS

Short Answer Question

List the expected serum range values for the following anticonvulsant medications:

1. Carbamazepine: _____

2. Diazapam: _____

3. Phenobarbital: _____

4. Phenytoin: _____

5. Valproic acid: _____

6. Primidone: _____

SAFETY *STAT!*

Review Question

The parents of a young child with a new diagnosis of a seizure disorder ask how they can prevent injury to their child if a seizure was to happen while they are at home or out in the community. To answer, the following tips are suggested: (*select all that apply*)

1. Maintain safety to the child's head by wearing a helmet, if ordered, at all times while awake
2. Administer anticonvulsant medication on time every day
3. Prevent dehydration
4. Keep child in front seat of car to maintain constant supervision
5. Remove furniture with sharp edges or glass surfaces
6. Begin home schooling

SAFETY *STAT!*

Labeling Exercise

Label Figures 29.2 and 29.3 as being decerebrate or decorticate posturing. In addition, for each illustration, state which part of the brain would be injured to cause this posturing.

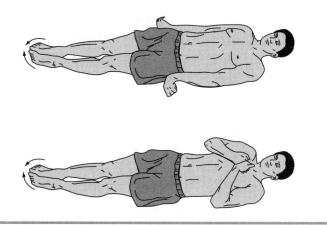

TYPES OF CHILDHOOD SEIZURES

Matching Exercise

_____ 1. Infantile spasms

_____ 2. Simple partial seizure

_____ 3. Complex partial seizure

_____ 4. Grand mal or tonic-clonic

_____ 5. Absence

_____ 6. Febrile

_____ 7. Status epilepticus

A. An uncommon, generalized seizure that presents between 3 months and 12 months of age, and that peaks at 4 to 8 months.

B. A type of disorder that progresses to other body sites with a loss of consciousness or an altered state of consciousness, and that is sometimes preceded by an aura. In infants, the child will demonstrate chewing, lip smacking, salivation, and excessive swallowing movements.

C. A type of seizure that only occurs in part of the child's brain. Symptoms depend on the location of electrical activity in brain; on average, this condition only lasts 10 to 25 seconds.

D. Rarely seen before 9 months of age or after the fifth birthday, this type of seizure is most commonly experienced during childhood and spontaneously remits without the use of specific anticonvulsant therapy.

E. A generalized seizure more often found in girls; it tends to develop after age 5. Often identified in a classroom setting as the child suddenly "checks out" and exhibits a blank stare, flickering eyelids, and a lack of general body movements.

F. A generalized dramatic seizure associated with an aura, a loss of consciousness, a shrill and piercing loud cry, and a tonic presentation followed by tonic-clonic movements of entire body alternating with relaxation of muscle. The child may experience pronounced saliva secretion, cyanosis due to apnea and a loss of bladder control, and sometimes with a loss of bowel sphincter control.

G. A type of continuous seizure that lasts longer than 30 minutes or the occurrence of serial seizures with no regained consciousness between them.

Child With a Sensory Impairment

30

Name: _____

Date: _____

Course: _____

Instructor: _____

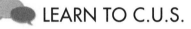 LEARN TO C.U.S.

Short Answer Question

A 2-year-old girl was admitted on the floor through a direct admit from a community pediatrician's office for severe retractable bacterial conjunctivitis. The child had been treated with three courses of antibiotics for the eye infection including two courses of antibacterial eye drops and one course of oral antibiotics. The child presents with very red, weepy eyes, and cellulitis extending from her left eye down her cheek. The nurse admitting the child notices a slight whitish glow from her left eye when the sunlight from the window hits her retina. The nurse is concerned that the child may have a more serious condition than a continuing conjunctivitis. Using the Learn to C.U.S. method of communication, how might the nurse report this concern to her charge nurse or hospitalist?

C: _____

U: _____

S: _____

THERAPEUTIC COMMUNICATION

Short Answer Questions

The pediatric nurse is working with a family in the emergency room. A young school-age child was brought in with facial burns from holding a faulty firecracker that exploded in the child's hands. The explosion burned his face and caused damage to his eyes. The plan of admitting the child in for more thorough diagnostics, antibiotics, wound care, and observation was just presented to the family. The mother is crying in grief, and the father is outwardly angry at the situation and is expressing his anger to the emergency room staff.

1. How might you approach this family to provide therapeutic communication?

   _____

   _____

   _____

2. Give three potential nursing diagnoses that pertain to this situation.

   1. _____

   2. _____

   3. _____

3. Provide a long-term goal pertaining to safety for this child's situation.

   Goal: _____

HEALTH PROMOTION

Table Completion

Complete the table by providing the definitions of the screening test and the required equipment.

Screening Test	Definition	Equipment Required for Screening
Lea symbol chart		
Unilateral cover test for infants or young children		
Corneal light reflex test		

TEAM WORKS

Short Answer Question

A toddler has experienced a trauma to her eyes with the penetration of a foreign object. The family is seeking medical attention at the local emergency room. What six health-care team members could you call to provide assistance to this family?

1. _____

2. _____

3. _____

4. _____

5. _____

6. _____

SAFETY *STAT!*

True or False Questions

1. _____ Conductive hearing loss is a form of hearing impairment where the inner ear has been affected by repeated otitis media causing scarring.

2. _____ The terms *deafness*, *hard of hearing*, and *hearing impairment* are all interchangeable.

3. _____ The term *enucleation* means to surgically remove the eye from the eye socket.

CULTURAL CONSIDERATIONS

Essay Question

A school nurse has been notified of a family whose young child is starting public school and will be a kindergartener. The child has recently been diagnosed with a severe sensory-neuro hearing loss requiring bilateral hearing aids. The kindergarten teacher has contacted the school nurse to report a conversation that took place during open house. The parents reported that they do not want the child to wear the hearing aid devices at school this first year, as they fear the child's peers will ridicule, bully, and/or socially isolate the child during his first year of public school. The child was brought to the open house without hearing devices on and although the child showed enthusiasm and was engaged with various stations set up in the classroom to introduce the children to art, puzzles, simple math, and music, the child did not talk to anyone and seemed content to be by himself. How would you respond to the teacher and what would you say to the family?

_____

_____

_____

_____

_____

CONCEPTUAL CORNERSTONE
True or False Questions

1. _____ A child's cognitive and social development may be at risk when there is the presence of a hearing or visual impairment, but only in the toddler, preschool, and school-age periods. Adolescents are able to adapt more readily and require less support.

2. _____ The family of a child with a viral otitis media will be offered the choice to administer antibiotics as viral otitis media often develops into a bacterial infection requiring aggressive antimicrobial medications.

REVIEW QUESTIONS

1. A father of a preschool child calls the pediatric clinic to discuss options associated with his child's hearing impairment. After seeing the pediatric hearing specialist, the father has questions about technology offered to promote school success. Which of the following forms of technology would benefit this child's age and development? (*select all that apply*)
   1. Cochlear implants
   2. Braille services
   3. Custom made hearing devices worn consistently during school and social interactions
   4. Computer keyboard adaptations
   5. Audiobooks
   6. Computer speech outputs

2. Which of the following is not considered an etiology of hearing impairment in children?
   1. Low Apgar scores during the neonatal period
   2. Anatomical malformation of head or neck
   3. Ototoxic drugs
   4. Family history of bacterial meningitis

3. An LVN is working in a community clinic serving low-income families. A family has told the pediatric health-care team that they cannot afford to purchase and maintain eyeglasses for their child. The nurse would be accurate to state that which national organization may be able to help provide glasses for their child?
   1. Rotary International
   2. Elks Club
   3. Soroptimist International
   4. Lyons Club International

SAFETY *STAT!*

Short Answer Question

In relation to the possibility of ototoxicity, which serum laboratory value associated with an ototoxic drug must be reported STAT if the values are too high?

SAFETY *STAT!*

Fill-in-the-Blank Questions

1. An LVN is attending a course to become certified in preschool vision screening. The course instructor describes that _____ % of all children have a visual disorder that requires further screening and follow-up care. Furthermore, the instructor describes how an estimated _____ to _____ children out of every 1,000 will have a visual impairment that prescription lenses cannot correct. These children may need surgical interventions to correct a visual impairment.

2. Acquired visual impairments are associated with a _____ _____ to the eyes, brain damage from _____ or _____ _____ _____ or a disease process whose consequence is an effect on the child's visual acuity.

PATIENT TEACHING GUIDELINES

Table Completion

Complete the table by providing the definitions to the eye disorders noted.

Amblyopia	
Astigmatism	
Cataracts	
Glaucoma	
Nystagmus	

Child With a Mental Health Condition

31

Name: _____

Date: _____

Course: _____

Instructor: _____

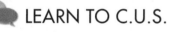 LEARN TO C.U.S.

Short Answer Question

A 13-year-old girl is admitted for pelvic inflammatory disease and is being treated by IV antibiotics. When talking with her, she tells the pediatric nurse that she is sexually active but does not want her parents to know. The nurse asks about condom use and whether or not she has access to contraceptives. She states no and says that she understands her current hospitalization is to treat a sexually transmitted disease. After talking with her for a while, she discloses that her father recently left her mother and her four younger siblings. She described her mother as a "drinker" and states she has had thoughts of ending her life. Using the C.U.S. method of communication, how might the pediatric nurse communicate his or her concerns about suicide risk to the health-care team?

C: _____

U: _____

S: _____

THERAPEUTIC COMMUNICATION

Short Answer Question

An autistic 10-year-old boy needs to have a deep intramuscular shot of a long-acting cephalosporin antibiotic prior to being discharged from the clinic. How might the pediatric nurse secure a team approach to be successful in the intervention while maintaining therapeutic communication for this school-age child with autism?

_____

_____

_____

REVIEW QUESTIONS

1. While documenting the effects of a newly ordered medication for attention deficit hyperactivity disorder (ADHD) the nurse is careful to monitor for which of the following side effects? (*select all that apply*)
   1. Restlessness
   2. Tremors
   3. Blurred vision
   4. Tachycardia
   5. Fever
   6. Headache

2. The father of a teenage girl with a diagnosis of schizophrenia asks about the best way to help her establish friendships with her peers. She is active in her church youth group, but has not established friendships outside of this community. Your best answer would be:
   1. "It is not realistic to expect that your daughter will establish friendships with her condition."
   2. "Having her older sibling with her will help her to meet kids around her age."
   3. "Having her interact with kids her age in her neighborhood might be a good start to establishing friendships close to home."
   4. "Children with schizophrenia can start relationships, but often due to behaviors, the friendships do not last long."

PATIENT TEACHING GUIDELINES

Short Answer Question

The mother of a child with depression is resistant to start her son on antidepressant medications. She expresses concerns about side effects, increased chance of suicide ideation, and risks of dependence. What can you say to the mother about antidepressant medications to help her feel more comfortable?

_____

_____

_____

SAFETY *STAT!*

True or False Questions

1. _____ When in the hospital, the parents of a child with ADHD might find controlling their child's behaviors especially difficult as their routines and familiar processes are thrown off.

2. _____ Using the term *mental illness* can be considered inadequate as there are often significant physical factors associated with the disorders.

3. _____ Mental health illnesses occur in childhood at an alarming rate in the United States. Current incidence rates are ~52%.

4. _____ Bullying is typically experienced in the school-age period and is associated with a child's lack of self-esteem.

5. _____ A child with anorexia nervosa will have a voluntary refusal to maintain a normal body weight at or above a minimally anticipated weight for their age, height, and size at 85% or less than expected.

SAFETY *STAT!*

Fill-in-the-Blank Question

Autism is considered one of a spectrum of conditions including Rett's syndrome and Asperger's syndrome. There is no known cause for autism but it is known to exist from the age of

_____. Autism can manifest with early symptoms in a child as young as

_____ _____. Autism is a condition that is

characterized by severe impairments in a child's _____ skills and

_____ _____.

TEAM WORKS

Matching Exercise

For a pediatric health-care team to be prepared to care for children with mental health concerns, consistent terminology must be used. Match the following key terms with the corresponding definitions.

_____ 1. Anorexia nervosa

_____ 2. Bulimia

_____ 3. Schizophrenia

_____ 4. Suicidal ideation

_____ 5. Suicidal thinking

A. A thought disorder marked by hallucinations, disorganized speech and behavior, and delusions.

B. When a child or teen is thinking about suicide but has no plan.

C. An eating disorder marked by weight loss, emaciation, disturbed body image, and an ongoing fear of weight gain.

D. When a child has recurrent episodes of binge eating followed by guilt, humiliation, shame, and then self-induced vomiting.

E. The thought process of considering suicide but without any physical attempts.

CULTURAL CONSIDERATIONS

Short Answer Question

The grandparents of a toddler recently diagnosed with autistic behaviors tell the parents that they should not disclose the mental health diagnosis to anyone else in the family, including the toddler's siblings. The parents ask the pediatric health-care team what they think should happen. What is your best response?

_____

_____

_____

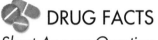 ## DRUG FACTS

Short Answer Question

An important concern for a family administering psychostimulant therapy to a child is to understand that a particular medication category and other substances are highly contraindicated while on ADHD medications. What is the medication category, what other substances should not be consumed, and what are the consequences of taking these contraindicated medications?

- Medication category: _____

- Other substances that should not be consumed: _____

_____

- Consequences of taking these contraindicated medications with ADHD medications:

_____

NURSING CARE PLAN

Short Answer Question

While caring for a teenager being seen at a community-based pediatric clinic, the LVN selects nursing diagnoses that are associated with the comprehensive and complex care required for children with the diagnosis of an eating disorder. State a nursing diagnosis and corresponding goal for this child.

_____

_____

Child With a Respiratory Condition

Name: _____

Date: _____

Course: _____

Instructor: _____

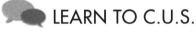 LEARN TO C.U.S.

Short Answer Question

As a nurse working at a public health clinic in a pediatric asthma clinic, you are assisting in the care of a child who presents with history of asthma. The child was released from the hospital just last week from an acute asthma exacerbation. You ask the child to show you how he uses his inhaler and you notice an inappropriate demonstration of the use of his inhaler. Using the C.U.S. method of communication, how would you express your concerns to the family?

C: _____

U: _____

S: _____

TEAM WORKS

Short Answer Question

The multidisciplinary team working together on an inpatient acute care pediatric unit is preparing for a child who has just been diagnosed with asthma to go home. The family, including both parents, grandmother, and older teenage sibling, have received asthma teaching, a list of medications to pick up from their local pharmacy, and follow-up visits with both the pediatric pulmonologist and the child's regular pediatrician. List the three categories of asthma medications that may be ordered for a child with asthma and why they would be ordered.

1. _____

2. _____

3. _____

CONCEPTUAL CORNERSTONE

Short Answer Question

State and define two concepts that relate to respiratory conditions during childhood.

1. _____

   Definition: _____

2. _____

   Definition: _____

PATIENT TEACHING GUIDELINES

Short Answer Question

Describe how you would explain, in detail, how to teach a family to lessen the probability of SIDS. Please provide eight topics for discussion.

1. _____

2. _____

3. _____

4. _____

5. _____

6. _____

7. _____

8. _____

TEAM WORKS

Table Completion

Define the following oxygen delivery systems.

Oxygen Delivery System	Definition
Oxygen tent	
Oxyhood	
Blow-by oxygen	
Nasal cannula	
Simple face mask	
Non-rebreather mask	
Venturi masks	

SAFETY *STAT!*

Review Questions

1. A preliminary diagnosis of cystic fibrosis has been made for a 4-year-old child. Which laboratory study should a pediatric nurse distinguish as confirming the diagnosis?
   1. Chest x-ray along with a pulmonary function test
   2. Sweat chloride test
   3. Blood culture and complete blood cell count
   4. Fecal fat collection
2. When an older infant has been determined to have cystic fibrosis, a concern the health-care team shares is that thick (tenacious) secretions can cause an obstruction in the respiratory tract. The nurse should observe for:
   1. Bronchopulmonary dysplasia
   2. Respiratory infections (pneumonia)
   3. Fibrosis in the lung tissue
   4. Need for more fluids to thin the secretions
3. A 3-year-old girl is diagnosed with croup. What is a sign of an impending respiratory emergency situation?
   1. She is crying and clinging to her mother.
   2. She refuses to take a sippy-cup of apple juice.
   3. She is experiencing a persistent cough.
   4. She is demonstrating restlessness.

4. The nurse is caring for a child who presents to the clinic with a concern of a diagnosis of metabolic acidosis. The child presents with a classic breathing pattern that demonstrates slow, deep, labored respirations often associated with metabolic acidosis. Which of the following breathing patterns most resembles the child's clinical presentation?
   1. Cheyne-Stokes breathing pattern
   2. Bradypnea breathing pattern
   3. Hyperventilation breathing pattern
   4. Kussmaul breathing pattern
5. The grandmother of a young preschool child who presents with epiglottitis tells the nurse she does not understand the definition of the medical diagnosis. The nurse would be most correct in stating that epiglottitis is:
   1. A form of croup.
   2. A life-threatening infection of the lung tissue.
   3. A swelling of the throat that can cause obstruction.
   4. An upper airway infection related to inflammation.

PATIENT TEACHING GUIDELINES

Short Answer Question

List 11 items that pose the greatest risk for aspiration and choking for young children.

1. _____
2. _____
3. _____
4. _____
5. _____
6. _____
7. _____
8. _____
9. _____
10. _____
11. _____

SHORT ANSWER QUESTIONS

1. What position would you expect a child to be in who is experiencing significant respiratory distress?

   _____

2. How would you define the color-coded zones representing a child's peak flow measurement?

   Green: _____

   Yellow: _____

   Red: _____

3. State the percentage of the child's peak flow for each color coding:

Green: _____

Yellow: _____

Red: _____

4. State, in general, what should be done for the child in each of the three color coding zones:

Green: _____

Yellow: _____

Red: _____

SAFETY *STAT!*

True or False Questions

1. _____ An apparent life-threatening event syndrome is a collection of diseases that usually occur in children under 1 year of age (infants).

2. _____ The symptoms may include cyanosis, apnea, coughing, gagging, and a change in muscle tone.

SAFETY *STAT!*

Matching Exercise

Match the key term to the corresponding definition.

_____ 1. Crepitus

_____ 2. Hemoptysis

_____ 3. Laryngitis

_____ 4. Cyanosis

_____ 5. Rhonchi

_____ 6. Stridor

A. A low-pitched adventitious breath sound when a mucus plug is within a large airway structure; a rattling sound that moves with coughing.

B. The presence of blood in respiratory secretions or mucus.

C. A high-pitched harsh sound that occurs during inspiration (often without the aid of a stethoscope), which denotes the presence of an obstruction in the upper airway.

D. A crackling sound heard while auscultating the lungs, such as with pneumonia.

E. Inflammation of the larynx or laryngeal mucosa and the vocal cords; characterized by hoarseness and aphonia (lost voice).

F. A blue, gray, slate-colored, or dark purple discoloration of the skin or mucous.

Child With a Cardiac Condition

Name: _____

Date: _____

Course: _____

Instructor: _____

 LEARN TO C.U.S.

Short Answer Question

A 2-year-old comes to visit the pediatric cardiology office to follow up with his cardiologist for a 4 week, postsurgical repair of a ventral septal defect. Both parents are with the child as they come into the reception area for a visit. Upon visual examination, the nursing staff sees that the child is flushed, sweaty, crying, and irritable. The nursing staff thinks the child might be ill and febrile. How might the nurses use the Learn to C.U.S. method of communication to report their initial visual findings to the medical team?

C: _____

U: _____

S: _____

CONCEPTUAL CORNERSTONE
Short Answer Question

Children with congenital cardiac conditions are at risk for the development of failure to thrive and low weight gain during infancy. Taking into consideration the concept of growth and development for an infant with a cardiac condition, what are three conditions that could cause an infant with a congenital heart defect to demonstrate lower weight gain?

1. _____

2. _____

3. _____

MATCHING EXERCISE

Match the correct cardiac defect description to the specific structural defect.

_____ 1. An opening in the septum between the left and right ventricles

_____ 2. A narrowing of the pulmonary artery or pulmonary valve

_____ 3. The pulmonary artery is connected to the left ventricle versus the right ventricle and the aorta is connected to the right ventricle versus the left ventricle

_____ 4. The tricuspid valve is completely obstructed

_____ 5. Incompletely developed mitral aortic valve, aorta, mitral valve, and left ventricle

_____ 6. A narrowing at or around the aortic valve

_____ 7. Four defects occurring simultaneously over-riding aorta, right ventricular hypertrophy, pulmonary stenosis, and ventricular septal defect

_____ 8. An opening in the septum that divides the left and right atria

_____ 9. A fetal shunt that connects the pulmonary artery and aorta and does not close after birth

_____ 10. A narrowing portion of the aorta typically located at or near the ductus arteriosis

A. Tetrology of Fallot

B. Coarctation of the aorta

C. Tricuspid atresia

D. Patent ductus arteriosis

E. Atrial septal defect

F. Ventricular septal defect

G. Hypoplastic left heart syndrome

H. Pulmonary stenosis

I. Aortic stenosis

J. Transposition of the great arteries

PATIENT TEACHING GUIDELINES
Cardiac Anatomy: Labeling Cardiac Structure and Blood Flow

The family of a neonate has just received the news that their newborn infant has been born with patent ductus arteriosus (PDA). The parents have asked you to draw a picture of the normal anatomy and circulation of their baby's heart so they can have a better understanding of the child's condition. In the spaces next to the illustrations found below, demonstrate your knowledge of cardiac anatomy, including circulation, by labeling the components of normal newborn circulation. Label the cardiac elements as noted below.

Label the ventricles and atria (Fig. 33.1):

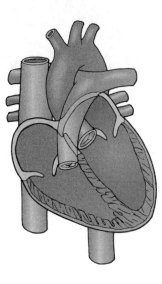

Label the vessels (Fig. 33.2):

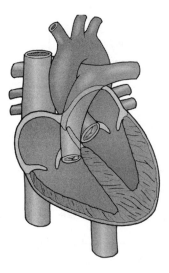

Label the direction of blood flow (Fig. 33.3):

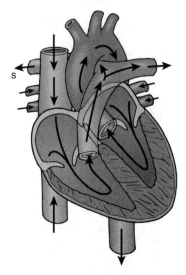

SAFETY *STAT!*

Review Question

While caring for an infant with a congenital heart defect, the nurse taking vital signs on the patient notices signs of poor perfusion that requires immediate notification of a primary health-care provider and immediate interventions. Which of the following are signs of poor perfusion? (*select all that apply*)

1. Cool extremities
2. Hypotension
3. Increased level of alertness
4. Weak or absent pulses
5. Prolonged capillary refill time greater than three sections
6. Increased urine output in response to fluid overload

SAFETY *STAT!*

True or False Questions

1. _____ Fetal blood flow is influenced by three pressures found in both the fetal lung and systemic system. These pressures include the low pressure of the systemic blood flow, the high pressures of the pulmonary blood flow, and the low pressure of the placental blood flow.

2. _____ Approximately 18 months after birth, the fetal shunts and shunt structures become ligaments.

3. _____ An accurate health history must be conducted by the cardiac pediatric primary care provider concerning symptoms associated with a congenital heart defect. If parents report cyanosis that worsens with activity and a heart murmur, these signs would be of concern.

PATIENT TEACHING GUIDELINES

Fill-in-the-Blank Question

While assisting the pediatric cardiac health-care team in helping parents of a newborn with a possible congenital heart defect understand the anatomy of the fetal heart in comparison to the newborn's heart, the cardiac clinic nurse hears the cardiologist say that the three fetal cardiovascular shunts are

_____, _____, and _____.

HEALTH PROMOTION
Short Answer Question

Infants and children with a cardiac defect may require the administration of digoxin. Specific safety guidelines must be given to the parents for accurate administration. Create a teaching plan for the parents of an infant in the cardiac clinic, who are learning about this new medication and who will be starting to give digoxin to their baby as a new home medication immediately. What are seven essential teaching points to reconfirm before leaving the clinic and filling the prescription?

1. _____

2. _____

3. _____

4. _____

5. _____

6. _____

7. _____

SAFETY *STAT!*
Fill-in-the-Blank Question

Do not give a child with a cardiac condition _____ without first consulting with the pediatric cardiac team and reporting the child's condition and symptoms. Indiscriminate use of

_____ can place the child at risk for complications associated with cardiac shunts and subsequent perfusion.

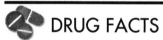 DRUG FACTS
Review Question

An infant is born with a congenital heart defect. In order to maintain adequate perfusion before the child undergoes a surgical procedure to repair the defect, a medication is administered to maintain cardiac vessel dilation and prevent clotting. The medication that is administered is:
1. Heparin
2. Surfactant
3. Prostaglandin
4. Indomethacin

CONCEPTUAL CORNERSTONE

Table Completion

An infant with a history of a congenital heart defect presents to their pediatric cardiologist's clinic because of concerns of poor feeding. The team conducts an assessment and determines the infant is demonstrating complications in perfusion.

Complete the following table about the differences between hypoxia and hypoxemia:

Hypoxia	Definition:	Clinical Evidence:
Hypoxemia	Definition:	Clinical Evidence:

Child With a Metabolic Condition

34

Name: _____

Date: _____

Course: _____

Instructor: _____

 LEARN TO C.U.S.

Short Answer Question

While discussing how the family is coping with the parents of a preschool-age child newly diagnosed with insulin-dependent (type 1) diabetes, the pediatric nurse asks about the child's adaptation to a lower sugar, carbohydrate-controlled diet. The parents describe how difficult this new way of eating is as there are four other children in the home all under 12 years old. The family states that the young child has difficulty not "sticking to the plan" and that because of the emotional impact of the new condition, they have not held her diet as close to the guidelines as they were taught. Upon further probing, the family states that they cannot plan a separate diet for their preschooler with diabetes mellitus (DM) and that because the condition is so new, they want to "give the child some time to adjust" while still eating the family's regular diet. The nurse realizes that the child's electronic chart is displaying higher than desired blood sugars and is concerned. How might the nurse use Learn to C.U.S. method of communication to state her concern?

C: _____

U: _____

S: _____

THERAPEUTIC COMMUNICATION

Short Answer Question

The young mother of a young infant has received the news that her child has a growth hormone deficiency. The child's growth plots on a standardized infant growth chart have displayed evidence of a consistent growth pattern under the third percentile. Laboratory analysis has demonstrated repeated evidence of low growth hormone. As the nurse is helping the mother and child settle into the examination room to be seen by an endocrinologist, the mother becomes tearful. How might you communicate support to the mother?

_____

_____

_____

_____

CONCEPTUAL CORNERSTONE: METABOLIC FUNCTION

Matching Exercise

Match the endocrine gland with the corresponding hormone:

_____ 1. Pancreas   A. Tyroxine

_____ 2. Pituitary gland   B. Calcitonin

_____ 3. Thyroid   C. Antidiuretic hormone

_____ 4. Testes   D. Follicle stimulating hormone

_____ 5. Ovary   E. Oxytocin

_____ 6. Adrenal   F. Thyroid stimulating hormone

                                     G. Adrenaline

                                     H. Testosterone

                                     I. Insulin

                                     J. Estrogen

SAFETY *STAT!*

True or False Questions

1. _____ Lipodystrophy is a complication of insulin injections where there is a change of subcutaneous fat under the skin, either atrophy or hypertrophy.

2. _____ The pituitary's anterior pituitary lobe is often referred as the "master" gland as it controls the release of the other hormones from the endocrine glands located throughout the body.

3. _____ Any signs of syndrome of inappropriate antidiuretic hormone (SIADH), including fluid retention, reduced urine output, or changes in the child's neurologic system, should be reported to the appropriate primary care provider.

TEAM WORKS

Short Answer Question

A young school-age child has just been discharged with a new diagnosis of type 1 diabetes from the hospital after an admission for diabetic ketoacidosis (DKA). The diagnosis requires a pediatric intensive care admission followed by 3 days on the inpatient pediatric ward. Many team members have provided support and care for this child and her family. List the various team members that could be involved in the care of a child newly diagnosed with insulin-dependent DM:

1. _____

2. _____

3. _____

4. _____

5. _____

6. _____

7. _____

8. _____

9. _____

10. _____

PATIENT TEACHING GUIDELINES

Table Completion

While preparing for the release of a family with a new diagnosis of insulin-dependent diabetes, the nurse prints out the required family education information about the insulins. Fill in the boxes with the definitions of each insulin type, the time of onset, and the duration of effectiveness.

Insulin	Type	Onset	Duration
Lispro (Humalog)			
Regular			
NPH/Lente			
Glargine (Lantus)			

SAFETY *STAT!*

Fill-in-the-Blank Questions

You are caring for a child who has come to the pediatric endocrinology clinic for a visit with their diabetes physician and the pediatric health-care team. The mother states that she has been using her own diabetic supplies for her child as she has lost the child's insurance and ran out of the child's supplies. The team expresses their concerns about her insurance and secures an appointment with the on-call social worker to provide assistance. The team then wants to review what the mother understands about the safe mixing or preparing of insulins, and asks the mother to state information about how best to mix insulins for administration safety. The following three topics are addressed. Please fill in the blanks:

1. Draw up the _____ insulin in an insulin syringe first, and then draw up the

   _____ insulin so that the clear insulin does not appear contaminated with the cloudy insulin if any enters the clear insulin vial.

2. Do not _____ any vials of insulin. Gently rotate the vial in your hand and treat it carefully. The amino acid chains can break with vigorous handling.

3. Do not _____ rapid-acting insulin Humalog Lispro (Humalog®) into the same syringe with a long-acting insulin Glargine (Lantus®).

SAFETY *STAT!*

Labeling Exercise

Label the following illustration (Fig. 34.1) with the glands of the endocrine system.

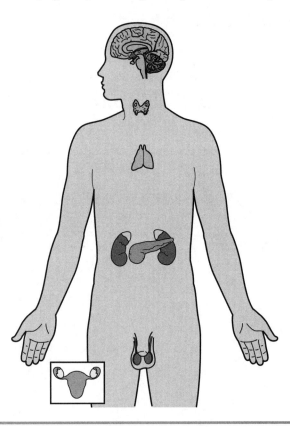

SAFETY *STAT!*

Short Answer Question

A child presents to the clinic for a follow-up exam after he was hospitalized for a significant head injury. The child presents with an unusual over production of clear, low specific gravity urine. The pediatric health-care team suspects the child is still symptomatic with diabetes insipidus (DI).

Differentiate between syndrome of inappropriate SIADH and DI.

SIADH: _____

DI: _____

TEAM WORKS: UNDERSTANDING HEMOGLOBIN A1c

Fill-in-the-Blank Question

Hemoglobin A1c is a measure of _____ _____.
It is followed as a routine check of the overall blood glucose level during the previous

_____ days.

SAFETY *STAT!*

Labeling Exercise

Label the illustration of an insulin syringe and note the chamber volume and total units in Figure 34.2.

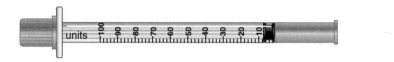

Child With a Musculoskeletal Condition

Name: _____

Date: _____

Course: _____

Instructor: _____

 LEARN TO C.U.S.

Short Answer Question

The family of a 2-year-old girl in Bryant's traction comes to the hospital to see their child every evening when the father gets off work. The visits are short but very meaningful for the family as they live more than a 1-hour drive from the hospital. The young girl is staying for at least 3 weeks during her recovery from a motor vehicle versus pedestrian accident. During the visit, the father asks if he can please hold his child as he did the night before. You become alarmed when you hear the traction had been removed for a period of time of the day before without the staff knowing. How might you use the Learn to C.U.S. method of communication to express your concerns to the father?

C: _____

U: _____

S: _____

THERAPEUTIC COMMUNICATION

Short Answer Question

The family of a newborn infant asks about the long-term effects of having congenital clubfoot. You ask the pediatric team to come and discuss the concerns being expressed by both parents about their infant daughter having bilateral clubfoot. What would the team say to the parents about the treatment and outcome of this condition?

_____

_____

_____

_____

CONCEPTUAL CORNERSTONE: DEVELOPMENT

Short Answer Question

List three activities for each of the developmental levels if a child is immobilized in traction:

Infant: _____

_____

_____

Toddler: _____

_____

_____

Preschool: _____

_____

_____

School-age child: _____

_____

_____

Adolescent: _____

_____

_____

TEAM WORKS

Short Answer Question

The family of a school-age child expressed concern about the child's time required in a state of immobilization for a healing compound (open) fracture of the femur. They are requesting to speak to the staff about a diet that will provide the nutrients needed for bone health. They also want to know about fiber to prevent constipation related to use of morphine for post-operative surgical pain as well as related to the child's state of immobility. You request that the dietician come to the pediatric unit and speak to the family with you. Describe ideas for food for bone health and foods for increased fiber:

Foods for bone health: _____

_____

_____

_____

Foods for increasing fiber: _____

_____

_____

_____

PATIENT TEACHING GUIDELINES

Short Answer Question

The parents of a child with a congenital unequal limb length who is going to have surgery asks about the differences between skeletal traction and skin traction. How would you define, describe, and differentiate these two forms of traction?

Skeletal traction: _____

_____

Skin traction: _____

_____

PATIENT TEACHING GUIDELINES

Review Questions

1. The family of a child born with congenital clubfoot has been prepared for the need of serial casting at 1 week then 2 week intervals. They have expressed concerns to the pediatric team about not wanting their young infant to be seen by extended family members with a cast on. Which of the following is the rationale behind this form of treatment?
   1. Casting is applied to the affected foot in order to stretch the ligaments and tendons.
   2. Casting is applied to prevent any further abnormal bone movement before surgery.
   3. Casting is required for at least 2 years to prevent the need for surgical repair.
   4. Casting is required after surgery is performed in the newborn period to prevent an injury that might cause the bone to move back into the clubfoot position.

2. When a child presents to the emergency room with a particular type of fracture, it causes the pediatric health-care team to suspect that the injury may have been intentionally caused. Which of the following fractures would cause the team to be suspicious?
   1. Greenstick fracture
   2. Spiral fracture
   3. Incomplete fracture
   4. Compound fracture

3. While discussing the results with the parents of their newborn's first assessment, the pediatrician explains to the family that the infant has a limited abduction of the right hip joint. The pediatric nurse then explains to the family that the newborn most likely has which of the following:
   1. Hairline fracture on the femoral head from birth trauma
   2. Congenital hip dysplasia
   3. Normal limited hip joint movement due to interutero positioning
   4. Birth trauma that will require a Pavlik's harness to correct

4. While reinforcing the medical treatment plan for a family whose newborn has talipes equinovarus, the nurse explains that the child will need serial casting at approximately which intervals?
   1. Every 2 weeks
   2. Every month
   3. Every week
   4. Intervals will depend on the child's progress

5. A family is being prepared by the pediatric nurse and member of the Child Life Team for a child who will be recovering from surgery and needing to be in traction for at least 1 month. The nurse knows that which of the following developmental stages experiences great stress while in traction due to the limited movement?
   1. Older infant who has learned to crawl well
   2. Toddler developmental stage
   3. Preschool child who is a magical thinker
   4. School-age child who needs the feelings of industry and accomplishment

SAFETY *STAT!*

True or False Questions

1. _____ A childhood fracture that involves the growth plate can cause temporary disruption in bone growth, but as the child enters early adolescence, the bone growth catches up and there are no long-term consequences to the injury.

2. _____ The five most common sites for a child to present with a fracture include the hand, elbow, clavicle, radius, skull, and orbital bone.

3. _____ Most pediatric orthopedists will tell a family to protect a child's fractured extremity for 2 to 4 weeks after a cast is removed.

PATIENT TEACHING GUIDELINES
Labeling Exercise

Children can present with a variety of traumatic injuries to their skeletal structure. Fractures are common across childhood. Label Figure 35.1 with the type of femur bone fractures: transverse, spiral, oblique, greenstick, and comminuted.

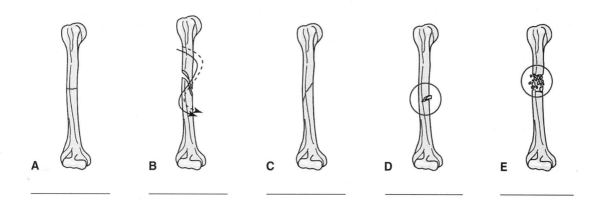

A _____   B _____   C _____   D _____   E _____

SAFETY *STAT!*
Review Questions

1. There are several hazards and complications to long-term traction. The following list represents examples of these concerns. Circle the correct items on the list that the pediatric nurse caring for a child in traction should be aware of: *(select all that apply)*
   1. Skin breakdown
   2. Boredom
   3. Decreased stimulation
   4. Pain and discomfort
   5. Respiratory congestion
   6. Diarrhea and gastrointestinal distress

2. Traction is used to provide realignment of the body part affected by injury or surgery. It is also used to provide a decrease in muscle spasms and provide immobilization. There are several types of components to traction that work together to help the child heal. Select all of the types of components to traction: *(select all that apply)*
   1. Friction
   2. Counter friction
   3. Counter traction
   4. Forward force

3. Significant extended post-operative pain has been known to delay wound healing in children. The pediatric nurse caring for a child who had a surgical manipulation of bone requires high doses of narcotic to achieve pain control. The nurse should administer the medication:
   1. As needed but right before the child requests the medication
   2. PRN
   3. When the parents begin to see the child having pain
   4. Around the clock

4. Osteogenesis imperfecta is a congenital condition caused by a defect of the gene that produces the precursor for collagen. The nurse understands that the condition is devastating, causes multiple skeletal fractures and is considered a:
   1. Recessive genetic disorder
   2. Dominant homogeneous disease
   3. Genetic disorder from faulty genes of one parent
   4. Dominant heterogeneous disease
5. While reinforcing information explained to the parents of a school-age child who is recently diagnosed with juvenile rheumatoid arthritis, the nurse explains the various medications that can be ordered. He tells the parents about each of the following medications: (*select all that apply*)
   1. Slower-acting antirheumatic drugs (SAARDs)
   2. Corticosteroids
   3. Acetaminophen
   4. Methotrexate
   5. Tumor necrosis factor inhibitors
   6. Salicylates

LABS & DIAGNOSTICS

Short Answer Question

While assessing a newborn for the presence of a shallow hip socket and the slipping of the femoral head within the acetabulum, the pediatrician performs two diagnostic procedures: an Ortolani's click maneuver and a Barlow's maneuver. Differentiate between these two.

Ortolani's click maneuver:

_____

Barlow's maneuver:

_____

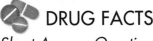 **DRUG FACTS**

Short Answer Question

Inflammation can be very damaging to the joints of a child who is diagnosed with juvenile rheumatoid arthritis. List the five classifications of drugs that are used to treat juvenile rheumatoid arthritis:

1. _____

2. _____

3. _____

4. _____

5. _____

Child With a Gastrointestinal Condition

36

Name: _____

Date: _____

Course: _____

Instructor: _____

 THERAPEUTIC COMMUNICATION: NURSING CARE
OF A CHILD WITH ENCOPRESIS

Short Answer Questions

While assisting the pediatric health-care team that is educating a family with a child with encopresis, a list of helpful ideas to promote the daily passage of adequate stool is prepared.
1. Define encopresis and then list eight helpful ideas that can assist the family to care for their child.
2. Search and list two reputable Web sites that can provide support for a family with a child with encopresis.

Definition of encopresis:

_____

_____

_____

_____

Ideas to help a family care for their child with encopresis:

1. _____

2. _____

3. _____

4. _____

5. _____

6. _____

7. _____

8. _____

Web site #1 _____

Web site #2 _____

CONCEPTUAL CORNERSTONE: ELIMINATION

Matching Exercise

Match the appropriate type of stool with the disorder

1. Hirschsprung's disease   A. Hard, formed
2. Intussusception   B. No change in stool
3. Appendicitis   C. Watery
4. Acute gastroenteritis   D. Possible diarrhea
5. Chronic constipation   E. Bloody stools
6. Celiac disease   F. Red currant jelly like
7. Crohn's disease   G. Thin ribbons

SHORT ANSWER QUESTION

Differentiate between the pathology and clinical presentation of Hirschsprung's disease from intussusception.

1. Hirschsprung's disease

_____

_____

_____

_____

2. Intussusception

_____

_____

_____

_____

SAFETY *STAT!*

Short Answer Question

List the order of a GI abdominal assessment using the five predominate assessment techniques, then give a rationale as to why this order is important with children:

1. _____

2. _____

3. _____

4. _____

5. _____

Rationale: _____

_____

_____

_____

LEARN TO C.U.S.

Short Answer Question

While caring for an older, school-aged child who is in the immediate post-operative period from surgery for a severely infected and ruptured appendix, the nurse notices that the child is displaying pain symptoms by slightly writhing in bed, pulling up his knees, grimacing, and being in a tearful state. He is trying to sit up and swing his legs over the side of the bed. He describes his pain as 8 out of 10 on the numerical pain scale, 1½ hours after the administration of intravenous morphine. The dose of morphine was appropriate for his weight per kilogram but does not seem to have the desired effect of post-operative pain management. Your goal is to attend to his pain and keep him in bed until he is comfortable and assisted to the bathroom as needed.

You decide that the hospitalist who is now following the child should be notified to report the continuation of pain after morphine and to discuss alternative pharmacological pain control measures. Using the Learn to C.U.S. model, describe how you would approach the hospitalist:

C: _____

U: _____

S: _____

TEAM WORKS AND PATIENT TEACHING GUIDELINES

Short Answer Question

The mother of a child newly diagnosed with Crohn's disease has asked you to help her understand dietary restrictions and suggestions to assist her child's condition. You decide to work with your pediatric health-care team and ask for a consultation with the dietary department. A nutritionist has come up to the floor to educate the family. What are five important topics to discuss with the family, the nutritionist, the child, and the health-care team?

1. _____

2. _____

3. _____

4. _____

5. _____

TEAM WORKS

Review Question

While caring for an older infant who was seen in the urgent care clinic for 3 days of diarrhea, the team determines the child has lost 7% of her body weight. She has a dry diaper and is refusing to drink from a bottle. What level of dehydration is she in?

1. Severe
2. Moderate
3. Critical
4. Mild

SAFETY *STAT!*

True or False Question

_____ The two most common types of dehydration associated with mild to moderate diarrhea are hypertonic dehydration and hypotonic dehydration.

SAFETY *STAT!*: CLINICAL PRESENTATION OF LEVELS OF DEHYDRATION

Table Completion

Mild
Moderate
Severe

NURSING CARE PLAN: Cleft Lip and Palate

Short Answer Question
List three priority nursing diagnoses for an infant with cleft lip and cleft palate.

1. _____

2. _____

3. _____

Child With a Genitourinary Condition 37

Name: _____

Date: _____

Course: _____

Instructor: _____

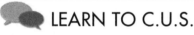 LEARN TO C.U.S.

Short Answer Question

A nurse is working with a multidisciplinary health-care team on a medical surgical pediatric unit of a large urban teaching hospital. A preschool child has been admitted with severely poor hygiene and underweight measurements. The nurse is concerned with her findings and wonders if this could be evidence of neglect. While she is assisting the child to the bathroom, the nurse discovers that the young child has a small amount of purulent discharge from either her vagina or her urethral opening. The child also complains of a burning sensation as she passes urine. Using the C.U.S. guidelines, how might the nurse phrase her concerns about this child to the charge nurse?

C: _____

U: _____

S: _____

TEAM WORKS

Short Answer Question

A pediatric nurse working at a large private pediatric clinic is providing care to a family of a newborn infant. While checking the patient in to the room, the mother expresses concern that her young male infant has an unusual appearing penis with a second "opening" at the base of the newborn's penis. The pediatric nurse inspects the child's genitalia and discovers there is potential anatomical anomaly.

Who should be immediately notified of this potential anatomical anomaly? Name three:

1. _____

2. _____

3. _____

 DRUG FACTS

Matching Exercise

Match the correct medical diagnosis with the medications administered to treat the genitourinary disorder.

_____ 1. Urinary tract
infection (UTI)

_____ 2. Glomerulonephritis

_____ 3. Nephrotic syndrome

_____ 4. Hypospadias

A. Diuretics

B. Antibiotics

C. 0.5% NS bolus

D. 25% albumin

E. Antifungal

F. Angiotensin-converting enzymes

G. Corticosteroids

H. Amoxicillin (Amoxil)

I. Sulfamethoxazole/trimethoprim (Bactrim, Septra)

CULTURAL CONSIDERATIONS

Essay Question

Conducting pelvic examinations on teenage girls can be influenced by the family's cultural background. Pelvic exams may be required as part of a complete physical exam if a teenage girl presents with a genitourinary condition. How might the nurse provide for a family and teenager whose cultural background does not permit her to be examined by a male in private without a family member there and when it is considered unacceptable to be unclothed?

_____

_____

_____

_____

SAFETY *STAT!*

Review Question

In order to be accurate on the intake and output of an infant who was admitted with a urinary tract infection, the nurse would measure urine output by which of the following methods?

1. Weigh the infant before and after voiding.
2. Insert an indwelling catheter to monitor urine output.
3. Send a urine specimen for specific gravity to measure the dilution of urine produced.
4. Weigh the infant's diaper.

CONCEPTUAL CORNERSTONE: ELIMINATION AND COMFORT

Short Answer Questions

A preschool-age child presents to the public health department pediatric clinic for irritability, fevers, lower abdominal pain, poor food and fluid intake, headache, and crying with urination. The mother tells the nurse that the child is now using the bathroom on her own and wiping herself after she urinates and defecates, no longer with parental assistance. Based on her presenting clinical symptoms, the health-care team suspects a urinary tract infection and decides to conduct a urinalysis with culture.

1. How is a urine specimen taken in a clinical environment?

_____

2. What are some tips the nurse can share with the family to push fluids for this young child who may be dehydrated?

_____

LABS & DIAGNOSTICS

Matching Exercise: Tests for Genitourinary Disorders

Match the diagnostic test with the corresponding test purpose.

_____ 1. Urinalysis

_____ 2. Urine culture and sensitivity

_____ 3. Specific gravity (SG)

_____ 4. Intravenous pyelogram

_____ 5. Voiding cystourethrogram (VCUG)

_____ 6. Blood urea nitrogen (BUN)

_____ 7. Blood creatinine

_____ 8. Creatinine clearance

A. Checks the kidney function by measuring the waste product of energy metabolism from muscle

B. Checks the bladder and surrounding structures during the process of voiding following the administration of contrast material (dye), which is instilled into the child's bladder to investigate the presence of reflux or strictures

C. Checked via machine to assess the concentration of urine

D. Checks the renal pelvic structures by radiography (x-ray) following the administration of an intravenously injected contrast material (dye)

E. BUN is a waste product of protein metabolism excreted via the kidneys

F. Checked for blood, glucose, ketones, protein, and pH

G. Collected for culture of bacteria or other infectious organisms and their sensitivity toward antibiotic therapy

H. Collected over time to measure the end product of energy metabolism from muscle

SAFETY *STAT!*

Short Answer Question

If a child weighs 34 pounds and a NSAID PO medication is ordered to reduce pain associated with a UTI and fever at 15 mg/kg, how much medication would she require? The medication comes as an over-the-counter liquid with 200 mg/10 mL. How many milliliters would the family need to prepare for each dose?

_____

_____

SAFETY *STAT!*

Short Answer Question

List the three types of dehydration and state the serum sodium associated with each type:

1. _____

2. _____

3. _____

NURSING CARE PLAN: Nursing Diagnoses

Short Answer Questions

Write two nursing diagnoses and two corresponding five-component goals for a young infant girl who is diagnosed with a urinary tract infection requiring a hospitalization for IV antibiotics. The five components of a goal are as follows: patient oriented, future oriented, realistic, measurable, and with a timeframe.

Nursing Dx: _____

Corresponding goal: _____

Nursing Dx: _____

Corresponding goal: _____

PATIENT TEACHING GUIDELINES

Short Answer Question

You are working with a registered nurse who is caring for a child with nephrotic syndrome. The child is ready for discharge and you hear the parents ask the nurse to describe what they should be looking for with a relapse of this condition. Describe four aspects of a relapse of nephrotic syndrome that should be taught by the members of the health-care team to parents of a child going home:

1. _____

2. _____

3. _____

4. _____

5. _____

SAFETY *STAT!*

Short Answer Question

While working for a home care company who serves chronically ill children, you have been assigned to care for a child who was hospitalized for their second relapse of nephrotic syndrome. The mother asks you what is the most appropriate amount of fluid her toddler can take per day: note that the child has been cleared for drinking fluids without restriction. To answer the mother, you calculate the fluid maintenance for this toddler who weighs 26 pounds.

Please provide your answer below.

Child With a Skin Condition

Name: _____

Date: _____

Course: _____

Instructor: _____

 LEARN TO C.U.S.

Short Answer Question

While assisting in the orientation of a new nurse to a busy inner-city pediatric health clinic, you are helping to show the new hire how to care for families in the clinic and how to implement safe practices. You note that although the new nurse performs his duties when bringing a family of a young child with possible varicella lesions back to one of the patient rooms, the new nurse does not follow any infectious disease precautions. You note that the child has several open, moist lesions on the skin on her face, neck, and arms. Taking into account that the child has not been diagnosed, and the lesions can be from many conditions, you feel concerned that no attempt to implement infection control has been done. How might you express your concerns to the newly hired nurse using the Learn to C.U.S. method of communication?

C: _____

U: _____

S: _____

SAFETY *STAT!*

Review Questions

1. When caring for children with severe and persistent itching, several nursing interventions can promote comfort. Which are appropriate? (*select all that apply*)
   1. Antihistamines
   2. Antipruritics
   3. Baking soda paste
   4. Heat from sun lamp
   5. Oatmeal paste
   6. Calamine lotions
   7. Baby wipe baths
2. Common skin disorders found in childhood are classified as all of the following *except:*
   1. Chemical
   2. Allergic
   3. Microbial
   4. Viral

THERAPEUTIC COMMUNICATION

Short Answer Question

The father of a preschool child is very upset that his son has been diagnosed with head lice. He has many questions about how the condition is passed between children and how he can prevent this from happening again. He states he does not understand how lice can be so readily passed in a preschool environment and is demanding to know what classroom conditions make lice infections so common. You calmly provide information about common classroom environmental factors that can contribute to lice infections. List four of these conditions:

1. _____

2. _____

3. _____

4. _____

PATIENT TEACHING GUIDELINES

Matching Exercise

Match the term with the corresponding definition.

1. Sumac
2. Pruritus
3. Urticaria
4. Contactant
5. Exanthem

A. Any type of a reaction or eruption that appears on the skin as opposed to a reaction or eruption that forms on mucus membranes.

B. A sensation of the skin that is burning or tingling that causes the child to itch, rub, or scratch.

C. Associated with allergic reactions and marked by multiple discrete areas of swelling on the skin (also known as wheals); can cause severe itching due to the associated secretion of vasoactive mediators from mast cells.

D. A shrub with the same active substance as poison ivy.

E. A substance that causes an allergic or sensitivity response when the substance is exposed to the skin.

TEAM WORKS

Short Answer Questions

1. A 14-year-old teen has been brought into the emergency department by paramedics after a significant burn. The team has assembled and you are to assist in the initial care of the child. After the team confirms that the child has a patent airway, has IV fluid and laboratory specimen access by the placement of two large bore IV needles, you take note the team is now going to use The Rule of Nines to estimate the distribution of burns in children. The young teen has burns on his entire left thigh (anterior and posterior), and left upper arm. How would you estimate the child's burn area to help confirm the team's estimation?

_____

_____

_____

2. While assisting a school nurse in a presentation to high school students who have infants under the age of one, the topic of safety is the overarching theme. You have been asked to present tips on how to prevent burns during the first year of life. List five tips you would provide:

1. _____

2. _____

3. _____

4. _____

5. _____

TEAM WORKS

Matching Exercise

In order to accurately document what a nurse observes when a lesion is discovered, match the lesions description with the lesion name by filling in the blanks with a corresponding letter from the descriptions:

_____ 1. Ulcer

_____ 2. Macule

_____ 3. Papule

_____ 4. Vesicle

_____ 5. Wheal

_____ 6. Pustule

A. Irregularly shaped lesions of cutaneous edema that look fluid filled, light center, and pale pink on the diameter.

B. A lesion that is filled with serous fluid, raised above the surface.

C. A flat, non-palpable lesion less than 1 cm in diameter.

D. An elevated, firm, palpable lesion that is less than 1 cm in diameter.

E. A loss of epidermis and dermis found in a concave shape in a variety of sizes.

F. A lesion that looks similar to a vesicle but is filled with pus.

SAFETY *STAT!*

True or False Questions

1. _____ Lyme disease, spread by deer tick bites, is difficult to diagnosis without a blood test because many children do not display the common Lyme disease rash.

2. _____ Petechiae is a serious rash associated with several systemic bacterial infections and can be found across childhood.

3. _____ The papillomavirus causes complications of acne for teenagers, especially during a female's menstrual cycle.

4. _____ Infants benefit from the oral administration of antihistamines for itching and pruritus caused by contact dermatitis.

5. _____ The most important distinguishing factor between contact dermatitis and a diaper rash from candidiasis is the presence of satellite lesions with yeast infections.

PATIENT TEACHING GUIDELINES

Short Answer Question

While confirming discharge instructions for a family taking a child home with a moderately sized open wound that requires dressing changes and antibacterial ointment spread into the base of the wound, you want to describe to the family optimal wound healing conditions. State four steps a family can recognize to help the child's wound optimally heal:

1. _____

2. _____

3. _____

4. _____

SAFETY *STAT!*

Review Questions

1. While speaking to the mother of a young child with a significant rash, the nurse would be correct in saying that which of the following assists the child in symptom management?
   1. Placement of cool washcloths on the skin
   2. Applying a thick layer of burn cream with a topical anesthetic
   3. Gently scraping off the sloughing tissue
   4. Wearing loose cotton clothing over the burn site
2. The treatment of minor sunburns includes all of the following *except:*
   1. Wearing snug fitting outfit to prevent the child from scratching
   2. Providing the child with clean cotton clothing
   3. Ensuring the child has synthetic materials to help wick moisture
   4. Placing soiled clothing in bleach soaks to kill bacteria

SAFETY *STAT!*

Short Answer Question

Who would you go see first and why?

Patient A: A teenager came to the urgent care clinic with a rash on his trunk that has raised red lesions streaking in various patterns. The teen said the rash is very itchy, has awakened and kept him up at night, and has been getting worse over the last 6 days. His mother confirmed that nothing they have tried has reduced the itching or the spread of the rash.

Patient B: A young child with a hand burn presents to the urgent care clinic. The front and the back of one hand looks bright red with some sloughing skin coming off the anterior and posterior sides. The child is crying inconsolably and the mother states that the older sibling spilled hot water from a teapot on to the child's hand.

_____

_____

_____

_____

_____

SAFETY *STAT!*

Table Completion

Complete the table, distinguishing between skin factors associated with a newborn and an infant related to their unique anatomy at their ages, and related to factors they experience due to environmental factors.

Newborn skin factors: Anatomy	1. 2.
Newborn skin factors: Environmental	1. 2.
Infant skin factors: Anatomy	1. 2.

Child With a Communicable Disease

Name: _____

Date: _____

Course: _____

Instructor: _____

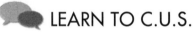 LEARN TO C.U.S.

Short Answer Question

While working on the pediatric unit, you notice that your colleague is answering a call light for the family of a child who is hospitalized for the administration of varicella immunoglobulins (IVIG) and is in strict isolation for open and wet-appearing varicella lesions. The child has a diagnosis of congenital neutropenia and is at high risk for complications associated with this childhood communicable disease. You see the nurse walk into the room without donning personal protective equipment. How might you use the C.U.S. method of communication to talk to her?

C: _____

U: _____

S: _____

SAFETY *STAT!*

Short Answer Questions

1. What type of isolation does a hospitalized child require for varicella lesions?

   _____

2. What personal protective equipment should he/she be putting on before entering the room of a child with open and wet-appearing varicella lesions?

   _____

   _____

   _____

3. Where can you find reputable information in a health-care setting and online concerning isolation techniques for various communicable diseases and the correct associated personal protective equipment?

   _____

   _____

   _____

THERAPEUTIC COMMUNICATION

Short Answer Questions

A parent is tearful as she explains to you that she feels responsible for the development of pertussis in her 7-week-old infant. She says the hospitalization is her fault as she did not believe in immunizations for her older preschool child and now feels guilty that her young infant and preschool child need to be treated with antibiotics for pertussis. She says the preschooler is home with the father and is on a long course of oral antibiotics. The infant is hospitalized for significant oxygen desaturations, persistent cough, and fever.

1. How would you address her immediate concerns?

   _____

   _____

   _____

2. What information would you like to see the team share with her to increase the understanding of childhood communicable diseases by improving adherence to an immunization schedule?

   _____

   _____

   _____

SAFETY *STAT!*

Review Questions

1. While working in a public health clinic, you encounter the family of a young child whose skin tests reveal that all four members of the family are positive for tuberculosis (TB). Treatment for tuberculosis includes:
   1. A 10 day course of oral antibacterial medications
   2. A 5 day course of intravenous tuberculin intravenous immunoglobulin
   3. A 3 day course of antineoplastic medication, such as methotrexate, for its resistant properties
   4. A 9 to 10 month course of oral anti-tuberculin medication
2. A tuberculosis infection in a child requires knowledge of transmission, incubation, and infection control. Tuberculosis is spread by:
   1. Droplets of mucus while coughing and sneezing
   2. Contagious airborne droplets while coughing, sneezing, or singing
   3. Contaminated surfaces where the child's body secretions have been in contact
   4. Contaminated hands after touching body secretions
3. When speaking with a family whose toddler was admitted with roseola, the nurse would be correct in stating that roseola is caused by:
   1. Streptococcal bacterial infection
   2. Herpes virus type 8 infection
   3. Staphylococcus bacterial infection
   4. Herpes virus type 6 infection

PATIENT TEACHING GUIDELINES

True or False Questions

1. _____ Young children with active TB are generally considered to be less infectious than adults with TB.

2. _____ A child's immune status will determine the symptom and severity of a TB infection.

3. _____ Children with viral infectious diseases need to have symptom control. To control fevers and discomfort, parents should administer aspirin.

PATIENT TEACHING GUIDELINES: RASH CARE

Short Answer Question

List eight ways that a family can provide comfort for a child who has a significant rash associated with a childhood communicable disease, such as varicella or measles?

1. _____
2. _____
3. _____
4. _____
5. _____
6. _____
7. _____
8. _____

TEAM WORKS

Short Answer Questions

While working at a large public health pediatric clinic, a family brings a child in with significant dehydration, weight loss, and a 1 week history of diarrhea. After taking vital signs and preparing the child to be seen by the nurse practitioner, you overhear the family talking about the diarrhea. The grandfather had just been hospitalized for 2 weeks with a history of diarrhea requiring antibiotics. You are concerned that the child might have been exposed to *Clostridium difficile*. You become concerned about the child needing isolation precautions while in the clinic.

1. Who do you need to tell about your concerns?

_____

_____

_____

2. What type of isolation should you implement while the child is in the clinic?

_____

_____

_____

3. What is the number one measure to prevent the spread of *C. difficile*?

_____

_____

_____

_____

SAFETY *STAT!*

Fill-in-the-Blank Question

Respiratory syncytial virus (RSV) is the most common cause of respiratory illness and lower respiratory tract infections in infants and children, and is a major cause of _____,

_____ and _____ _____. In

the adult population, RSV often causes _____ _____.
The effect on infants in children can be far more significant. At particular risk for severe respiratory

complications from RSV infection are _____ and especially

_____ _____.

SAFETY *STAT!*

Short Answer Question

Serious complications of varicella are rare but can occur. List nine possible complications of a severe varicella infection:

1. _____

2. _____

3. _____

4. _____

5. _____

6. _____

7. _____

8. _____

9. _____

TEAM WORKS

Short Answer Question

What are two important measures to prevent the spread of infection from a hospitalized child or a child seen in clinic who has a confirmed diagnosis of a childhood communicable disease?

1. _____

2. _____

PATIENT TEACHING GUIDELINES

Matching Exercise

1. Endemic

2. Epidemic

3. Communicable

A. Capable of being transmitted from one individual to another.

B. The presence, or prevalence, of a disease within a particular region. May be natural presence within a particular place, such as threadworms are endemic to tropical areas.

C. The presence, or prevalence, of a disease within a widespread geographical area. Typically refers to a rapid spread or an increased occurrence of a disease within a widespread geographical area.

Child With an Oncological or Hematological Condition

40

Name: _____

Date: _____

Course: _____

Instructor: _____

CONCEPTUAL CORNERSTONE: CELLULAR REGULATION

True or False Questions

1. _____ Children with a medical diagnosis of beta thalassemia minor will be required to receive blood transfusions on a regular basis throughout the rest of their lives.

2. _____ A child with severe anemia caused by the over-consumption of milk should be restricted to 32 ounces of milk intake daily.

3. _____ Families who worship in the faith of Jehovah's Witnesses avoid the transfusion of blood products.

CONCEPTUAL CORNERSTONE: CELLULAR REGULATION

Fill-in-the-Blank Questions

1. The most commonly transfused blood product for children with a hematology/oncology disorder is

_____ _____ _____

_____ .

2. A trigger often causes a child with sickle cell anemia to experience a sickle cell episode. These episodes lead to the bone marrow producing rigid sickle-shaped RBCs, which increases

_____ _____ and causes

_____ _____ due to the obstructed blood

flow.

CASE STUDY: TEAM WORKS

Short Answer Question

Frankie is a 14-year-old who has had a diagnosis of leukemia. He now suffers from severe anemia from the side effects of the chemotherapy. The Oncology Health Care Team has assembled for their weekly patient conference and prioritizes Frankie's ongoing anemia. Describe the six ways in which anemia can develop.

1. _____

2. _____

3. _____

4. _____

5. _____

6. _____

CONCEPTUAL CORNERSTONE

Essay Question

The nurses caring for a young child receiving high-dose induction chemotherapy have determined that few members of the health-care team (including housekeeping, dietary, and facilities) are maintaining safety by adhering to strict neutropenic precautions while entering the child's room and interacting with the family. The nurses decide to investigate the best current practices on neutropenic precautions. They have decided that they "Have a concern, are uncomfortable with the safety issue of protecting the child's compromised immunity, and want to create a safety net."

Describe 10 neutropenic precautions that can be implemented to protect a child during a neutropenic state caused by the effects of chemotherapy.

1. _____

2. _____

3. _____

4. _____

5. _____

6. _____

7. _____

8. _____

9. _____

10. _____

💬 THERAPEUTIC COMMUNICATION

Short Answer Question

A child is brought into a children's hospital outpatient transfusion center with severe anemia. The family is speaking to the charge nurse about the concerns they have regarding their young child's need to have a first-time blood transfusion; they have read about the potential side effects and reactions. While speaking to the family, the nurse covers the following potential reactions to transfused blood products so that the family has complete informed consent:

_____

_____

_____

SHORT ANSWER QUESTIONS

Symptoms of Blood Transfusion Reactions

Describe the symptoms associated with the following blood transfusion reactions:

1. Febrile:

_____

_____

_____

2. Urticaria:

_____

_____

_____

3. Hemolytic responses:

_____

_____

_____

4. Alloimmunization:

_____

_____

_____

5. Septic shock:

_____

_____

_____

6. Circulatory overload:

_____

_____

_____

SHORT ANSWER QUESTIONS
Interventions for Blood Transfusion Reactions

Describe the interventions for each of the following blood transfusion reactions:

1. Febrile:

2. Urticaria:

3. Hemolytic responses:

4. Alloimmunization:

5. Septic shock:

6. Circulatory overload:

SHORT ANSWER QUESTIONS

1. Define alopecia: _____

2. Describe how you would teach a teenager about chemotherapy-induced alopecia:

REVIEW QUESTIONS

Mr. and Mrs. Parker are speaking to the pediatric health-care team members about their infant son's diagnosis of sickle cell anemia.

1. Which of the following statements, if stated by the parents, would require the team to offer more teaching on the pathology of this condition?
   1. Sickle cell anemia is caused by a reaction to exposure to an environmental toxin.
   2. Hemoglobin S sickles in the situations where the child experiences hypoxia.
   3. Sickle cell anemia is associated with a gene responsible for the production of abnormal hemoglobin.
   4. Sickle cell anemia is found in persons of Mediterranean and African ancestry.

2. Which of the following laboratory tests and diagnostics are associated with the care of a child with leukemia receiving treatment? (*select all that apply*)
   1. Absolute neutrophil count
   2. Reticulocyte count
   3. White blood cell count
   4. Erythrocyte sedimentation rate
   5. Platelet count

MATCHING EXERCISE

Match the four common types of sickle cell anemia (SCA) crisis situations with the correct definitions.

1. Vaso-occlusive crisis

2. Aplastic anemia crisis

3. Sequestration crisis

4. Hyperhemolytic crisis

A. This type of SCA crisis is caused by an increasing rate of RBC destruction, which leads to severe anemia and a state of jaundice.

B. This type of SCA crisis lasts up to 6 days and presents with severe pain in the joints, bones, and abdomen, and with swollen joints, feet, and hands. The child may experience visual disturbances.

C. This type of SCA crisis is caused by large quantities of blood that collect and pool in the child's spleen and liver, causing tachycardia, weakness, and dyspnea. It may lead to shock as the vascular volume of the child's blood decreases.

D. This is a form of extreme anemia caused by the severe destruction and lack of production of the child's sickle-shaped RBCs.

Bonus Chapters

Introduction to QSEN

1

Name: _____

Date: _____

Course: _____

Instructor: _____

💬 LEARN TO C.U.S.

Short Answer Question

A 15 y.o. patient, Zoya, is being seen in the surgical clinic as a follow-up visit after being hospitalized for 5 days with acute appendicitis. While taking her vital signs and checking her in, you note that she exhibits signs of drug use and clinical depression. During one tearful exchange, Zoya disclosed suicidal thoughts brought on by grief from the recent suicide of a friend. Zoya's parents are dismissive of Zoya's fragile emotional state. The physician is unaware of these issues. Using the Quality and Safety in Nursing Education (QSEN) competencies of effective communication, teamwork, and safety, how might you approach your clinic's charge nurse to report the above situation and provide safety for this teenage girl? Use the Learn to C.U.S. method of communication:

C: _____

U: _____

S: _____

SAFETY *STAT!*

Short Answer Question

The Institute of Medicine (IOM) stated that improvements are required to address the flaws in the current health-care system as a whole. A new 21st century health-care system was envisioned that would include the following six imperatives:

1. _____

2. _____

3. _____

4. _____

5. _____

6. _____

THERAPEUTIC COMMUNICATION

Short Answer Question

The QSEN initiative addressed this need by outlining the skill sets required by nurses in this 21st century workforce. These skill sets include competencies in six areas. List the six areas of the QSEN initiative:

1. _____

2. _____

3. _____

4. _____

5. _____

6. _____

TEAM WORKS

Review Question

The QSEN initiative was created partially in response to the IOM report on medical errors in health care. The IOM is a powerful and prominent voice that acts under congressional charter to advise which of the following organizations?
1. The federal government on matters pertaining to public health.
2. State and local branches of private and public hospitals.
3. Schools of nursing to create safety-based curriculum.
4. The international community to create world standards.

CULTURAL CONSIDERATIONS

Short Answer Question

In the Learn to C.U.S. case about Zoya, you learn that her parents are Muslim, although Zoya herself has not embraced her parents' faith. How might this information influence how the pediatric health-care team comes together to offer the QSEN competency of Patient and Family-Centered Care and secure safety for this teen?

_____

_____

_____

SAFETY *STAT!*

True or False Questions

1. _____ The report published by the IOM titled, *"To Err is Human"* stated that more than 98,000 Americans die each year as a result of medical errors.

2. _____ According to the Committee on the Robert Wood Johnson Foundation Initiative on the Future of Nursing (2011), nurses are the largest segment of the health-care workforce, and their skills and availability can directly affect quality, safety, and efficiency.

TEAM WORKS

Essay Question

You have been requested by your clinical faculty to make a small presentation to your classmates based on the QSEN competencies. You are asked to determine the five most common causes of preventable deaths in children on a national level. Locate a nationally recognized source of data to determine the top five. Craft a fictional 30-second radio announcement in which you educate parents about the safety issues related to both the risks and the strategies for preventing one of the five most common causes of preventable deaths.

_____

_____

_____

_____

_____

_____

_____

TEAM WORKS

Short Answer Question

Define the term *just culture* as it relates to reporting medical errors.

Cultural Competency in Maternity and Pediatric Care

2

Name: _____

Date: _____

Course: _____

Instructor: _____

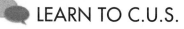 LEARN TO C.U.S.

Short Answer Question

You are working with a team of health-care providers at a health fair held at a local community center providing basic screening for families. Families have lined up with their children to receive blood pressure screening, glucose testing, immunizations, healthy eating information, and body mass index (BMI) measurements. While assisting with the team, you notice a verbal exchange between a mother and a nurse. The mother has described how her religious/cultural group forbids her from accepting childhood immunizations on the grounds that "the immunizations are meant to control children and are very harmful." The nurse is arguing loudly with the mother saying "her type" is causing epidemics of pertussis and measles around the nation. You become concerned, as the interchange is becoming hostile and the two families closest to the tables walk away with their children. Use the Learn to C.U.S. method of communication to express your concerns to the nurse and mother.

C: _____

U: _____

S: _____

💬 THERAPEUTIC COMMUNICATION

True or False Question

_____ Inclusivity is the fact or policy of excluding members or participants on the grounds of gender, race, class, sexuality, disability, or other factors.

TEAM WORKS

Fill-in-the-Blank Question

Within the context of health-care environments, _____ exists among persons or patients seeking care, and among the health professionals providing care.

TEAM WORKS

Review Question

While attending a conference offered by the local public health clinic on how to care for diverse families, the presenter states that the definition of cultural awareness is which of the following?
1. Providing care where all people are treated the same regardless of cultural diversity.
2. Understanding that people differ and require health providers of the same ethnicity.
3. Developing sensitivity and awareness of another ethnic group.
4. Becoming aware of the demographics of one's community.

💬 THERAPEUTIC COMMUNICATION

Matching Exercise

_____ 1. Diversity

_____ 2. Cultural sensitivity

_____ 3. Cultural awareness

_____ 4. Ethnicity

_____ 5. Health literacy

A. The degree to which individuals have the capacity to obtain, process, and understand basic health information and services needed to make appropriate health decisions.

B. The perception of oneself and a sense of belonging to a particular ethnic group, or to more than one group. This term includes commitment to cultural customs and rituals. It is not the same as physical traits associated with race (skin or eye color, or hair) or those related to a geographical origin.

C. Differences in race, ethnicity, national origin, religion, age, gender, sexual orientation, ability or disability, social and economic status or class, education, and related attributes of groups of people in society.

D. Developing sensitivity and awareness of another ethnic group.

E. The experience when neutral language, both verbal and not verbal, is used in a way that reflects sensitivity and appreciation for the diversity of another.

TEAM WORKS

True or False Question

_____ National Standards for Culturally and Linguistically Appropriate Services in Health Care (CLAS) is a set of collective standards that include recommendations to guide and inform culturally appropriate health services for hospitals, clinics, and health services.

SAFETY *STAT!*

Fill-in-the-Blank Question

As global migration has an impact on _____ _____ upon individuals and families as they transition from one culture to another, the same can be said of global migration and political factors. Information about health care within the political context people have experienced as they move from one place to another adds another level of understanding in

_____ and decision making.

THERAPEUTIC COMMUNICATION

Review Question

The term *culture* is important for nurses to understand the needs of children and their families. Which of the following components make up the definition of culture? (*select all that apply*)
1. Foods and food preparation
2. Dress
3. Language
4. Educational level
5. Customs
6. Beliefs

SAFETY *STAT!*

Short Answer Question

The concept of health-care disparities across populations is concerning. Give two examples of the consequences that health-care disparities cause for people in America.

Consequence #1: _____

Consequence #2: _____

TEAM WORKS

Short Answer Question

Cultural assessment tools offer a guideline for communication, planning, implementation, and evaluation of care. Each health-care organization or setting may have assessment tools unique to the demographics of a particular location. A culturally appropriate assessment takes into consideration at least five factors. State five factors:

1. _____

2. _____

3. _____

4. _____

5. _____

SAFETY *STAT!*

True or False Question

_____ According to the U.S. Department of Health and Human Services investigation on communication and ethnicity, Blacks, American Indians, and Alaska Natives reported poor communication with doctors, and patients who spoke Spanish at home reported higher poor communication with nurses than white patients.

Women's Health Promotion Across the Life Span

Name: _____

Date: _____

Course: _____

Instructor: _____

REVIEW QUESTIONS

1. A nurse notices that a patient has several flesh-colored warts on her perineal area. The nurse suspects that the patient has become infected with:
   1. Gonorrhea
   2. Human papillomavirus (HPV)
   3. Herpesvirus
   4. Syphilis

2. A nurse is discussing diaphragm use with a postpartum patient. The patient demonstrates understanding of correct use of a diaphragm when she states:
   1. "I can use the same diaphragm that I used before I gave birth."
   2. "I must leave it in place for 6 hours after I have sex."
   3. "I'm glad that I don't need spermicides."
   4. "A diaphragm protects me from sexually transmitted infections."

3. A 17-year-old woman who had unprotected sex 12 hours ago has entered the clinic asking for assistance because she is concerned about her pregnancy risk. Which of the following statements by the nurse is appropriate?
   1. "Because you're only 17, we can't help you."
   2. "It's too late to prevent a pregnancy."
   3. "You should have insisted that he use a condom."
   4. "Plan B is available to prevent a pregnancy."

4. The nurse is aware that hormone replacement therapy is effective for:
   1. Women with a history of breast cancer.
   2. Women with coronary artery disease.
   3. Women with pelvic floor weakness.
   4. Women with severe menopausal symptoms.

5. A teenager is talking to the nurse and says, "Every month right before my period, I get irritable. No one wants to be around me. I feel bloated and just want to eat chips." The nurse suspects that the teenager has the symptoms of:
   1. Perimenopause
   2. Pelvic inflammatory disorder
   3. Premenstrual syndrome
   4. Premenstrual dysphoric syndrome

6. A nurse is giving discharge instructions to a man who just underwent a vasectomy. Which statement should be included in the plan of care? (*select all that apply*)
   1. "You will need to use another form of birth control for 3 months."
   2. "If you change your mind, vasectomies are easy to reverse."
   3. "You will need to be off work for at least 6 weeks."
   4. "You should bring in a semen specimen for testing in about 3 months."
   5. "You need to measure your urinary output, just to make sure there are no complications."

7. A woman states that she "feels funny touching her private parts." Which form of contraception would not be appropriate for her?
   1. The contraceptive implant
   2. Oral contraceptives
   3. Condoms
   4. Cervical cap

8. A woman calls the clinic and states that she is having a stinky green vaginal discharge and itching of her labia. The nurse makes an appointment for the patient because the nurse suspects:
   1. Contact dermatitis
   2. Syphilis
   3. Vulvovaginitis
   4. Trichomonas

9. A woman reports that she has blisters and burning in her perineal area. The nurse suspects:
   1. Human papilloma virus
   2. Herpesvirus
   3. Syphilis
   4. Gonorrhea

10. A nurse is discussing pelvic inflammatory disease (PID) with a patient. The patient indicates that she needs more teaching when she says:
    1. PID can occur after an untreated sexually transmitted infection.
    2. PID has no major complications.
    3. PID requires antibiotic therapy.
    4. PID can require a hospitalization.

TRUE OR FALSE QUESTIONS

1. _____ A DEXA (dual energy x-ray absortiometry) scan for osteoporosis should be done at age 75.

2. _____ Toxic shock syndrome is associated with tampon use.

3. _____ Contact dermatitis can be caused by vaginal and perineal cleansing products.

4. _____ HPV puts a woman at risk for AIDS.

5. _____ Primary amenorrhea is the failure of menses to occur by age 13.

6. _____ Women with a history of venous thrombosis are not good candidates for oral contraceptives.

7. _____ Secondary amenorrhea can be due to extreme weight loss.

8. _____ Endometriosis can cause infertility.

9. _____ Spermicides should be left in the vagina for 30 minutes after intercourse.

10. _____ A woman with a history of breast cancer should not use hormonal contraceptives.

SAFETY *STAT!*

Short Answer Question

Complete the acronym ACHES to remember the warning signs that women should report when taking oral contraceptives.

A = _____

C = _____

H = _____

E = _____

S = _____

MATCHING EXERCISE

_____ 1. Amenorrhea

_____ 2. Dysmenorrhea

_____ 3. Endometriosis

_____ 4. Fibroids

_____ 5. Hirsutism

_____ 6. Hysteroscopy

_____ 7. Leiomyoma

_____ 8. Myomas

_____ 9. Osteoporosis

_____ 10. Vulvovaginitis

A. Benign tumor of smooth muscle.

B. Infection of the vagina and vulva.

C. A tumor containing muscle tissue.

D. A condition in which the bones become thin and fragile.

E. Painful menstrual periods.

F. Abnormal growth of hair on the face and body, particularly in women.

G. A lighted scope is placed through the cervix into the uterus to visualize the uterine cavity.

H. The absence of a menstrual period.

I. Benign tumors in the uterus.

J. A condition in which uterine tissue is growing outside the uterus.

SHORT ANSWER QUESTIONS

1. _____ amenorrhea is failure of menses to start by age 16.

2. A condition in which uterine tissue grows outside the uterus is called

   _____.

3. Pain that occurs with ovulation is called _____.

4. List three medications that may be used to treat premenstrual syndrome (PMS).

1. _____

2. _____

3. _____

5. To decrease fluid retention and bloating in PMS, a woman should avoid

_____.

6. The birth control method that prevents the transmission of sexually transmitted disease is the

_____.

7. The _____ _____ is the best choice of an oral hormonal contraceptive for women who are breastfeeding.

8. List two disadvantages of injected depot medroxyprogesterone acetate for hormonal contraception.

1. _____

2. _____

9. List two risk factors for infertility.

1. _____

2. _____

10. A _____ is an x-ray with dye to visualize the female reproductive organs.

11. List two possible causes of male infertility.

1. _____

2. _____

12. List two possible causes of female infertility.

1. _____

2. _____

13. Vasomotor symptoms of menopause include _____ and

_____ _____.

14. List three nursing interventions to manage the symptoms of menopause.

1. _____

2. _____

3. _____

15. A _____ cyst occurs when the follicle cyst does not open to release the egg.

TABLE COMPLETION

Complete the table on pelvic floor disorders.

Disorder	Description	Symptoms
Cystocele		
Rectocele		
Prolapse of the uterus		
Prolapse of the vagina		

THERAPEUTIC COMMUNICATION

Short Answer Question

Utilizing therapeutic communication techniques, formulate some statements and questions you could use when discussing contraception with a teenager.

HEALTH PROMOTION

Short Answer Questions

1. Identify three methods to reduce the risk of transmission of sexually transmitted infections (STIs).

2. Identify three ways a woman can reduce her chance of getting toxic shock syndrome.

_____

_____

_____

3. Identify three ways a woman can reduce her chance of getting pelvic inflammatory disease.

_____

_____

_____

POST-CONFERENCE QUESTIONS AND ACTIVITIES

1. Find an online resource, such as YouTube, and find a video about contraceptives. Critique it for accuracy and share your report at post-conference.

2. Find an online resource, such as YouTube, and find a video about sexually transmitted infections. Critique it for accuracy and share your report at post-conference.

SAFETY STAT!

Short Answer Questions

1. A woman at the family planning clinic is interested in obtaining an intrauterine contraceptive device (IUD). What question should the nurse ask to determine whether it is a safe method of contraception for her?
2. Another woman at the family planning clinic is interested in an oral contraceptive. What questions should the nurse ask her to determine whether the oral contraceptive is a safe method for her?

Adapting to Chronic Illness and Supporting the Family Unit

4

Name: _____

Date: _____

Course: _____

Instructor: _____

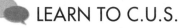 **LEARN TO C.U.S.**

Short Answer Question

The mother of a child with cerebral palsy (CP) needs to learn how to give her child anticonvulsants via his new percutaneous endoscopic gastrostomy (PEG) tube as the child has been demonstrating increasing choking with oral medications. Because the child is considered at risk for aspiration, the mother needs to be taught how to draw up the medications and administer the medication flush. The mother has not been seen at the hospital for 2 days and refused to believe the doctor when he said that her son will need daily anticonvulsants for his chronic illness, saying that the child's symptoms were not seizure activity, but rather spasms from his history of CP. The nurse becomes concerned when the team discusses the impending discharge and the mother has not been seen. How might you word your concerns to the team?

C: _____

U: _____

S: _____

THERAPEUTIC COMMUNICATION

Short Answer Question

The father of a young child newly diagnosed with a life-threatening respiratory illness who is now chronically ill with residual respiratory insufficiency becomes very angry while his daughter is hospitalized. The father feels that the hospitalist on duty does not know his daughter sufficiently and is ordering invasive diagnostic exams that he perceives will cause his daughter discomfort and fear. He becomes angry and begins to pace the halls visibly upset and loudly, shouting demands for a pediatrician to come who knows his daughter's medical history. Which of the following answers would be the best response a care professional could say to the father?

1. "Could you please go into your daughter's room? Your behavior is frightening the other patients and families."
2. "I can understand that you are feeling anger right now. It must be frustrating to work with a team that does not know your daughter's medical history as well as you do."
3. "Can we go into the family room? I will call the nursing supervisor and see if he has time to come and talk to you."
4. "This is highly inappropriate behavior on the pediatric floor, sir. If you do not calm down I will need to call security."

Give a rationale for your answer:

_____

_____

_____

TEAM WORKS

True or False Questions

1. _____ The role of the Child Life Specialist in caring for siblings of a child with a chronic illness is to provide supervision, distraction, and education.

2. _____ Toddlers understand the concept of cause and effect, therefore they can understand the process of death as being permanent.

CONCEPTUAL CORNERSTONE

Short Answer Question

A teenage child diagnosed 12 years ago with cystic fibrosis has been admitted for the fourth time in the last 6 months with pneumonia. Her lungs have demonstrated severe disease and she has a persistent wet cough with the inability to adequately clear her thick pulmonary secretions. On admission, she presents with oxygen saturations of 86% to 88%, oxygen dependency, fevers, respiratory distress, tachypnea, tachycardia, extreme fatigue, and dehydration. She is very quiet and looks despondent. Keeping in mind the concept of safety, define what is meant by the following terms related to exacerbations of a chronic illness:

1. Aggravation of symptoms: _____

2. Relapse of an acute phase: _____

PATIENT TEACHING GUIDELINES

Matching Exercise

Match the key term with the corresponding definition.

_____ 1. Chronicity

_____ 2. Chronic illness

_____ 3. Normalcy

_____ 4. Technology dependent

_____ 5. Special needs

A. A child's state when he or she has a functional limitation or disability that requires special assistance; this construct can pertain to autism, sensory impairment, impaired mobility, technology dependency, or an emotional/psychological disorder.

B. Pertaining to a condition lasting a long time.

C. The dependence on a medical device and/or skill to maintain health and wellness.

D. The movement toward being normal in one's life; pertains to attaining normal standards in one's life when faced with chronic illness, disability, or impairment.

E. An illness that lasts a long period of time and significantly affects a person's functioning for at least 3 months of each year.

SAFETY *STAT!*

True or False Questions

1. _____ In terms of safety, the goal of care for a child with a chronic illness is to minimize autonomy as the child requires dependence on parents and others to provide technology and specialized skills.

2. _____ The premise behind a diagnosis of a chronic illness is that the child will receive treatments that will cure the child of the chronic ailment so that in adulthood they can expect to be free of the chronic condition.

TEAM WORKS

Review Question

Although no national registries exist to document the exact number of chronically ill children, many organizations exist that can provide information on various chronic illnesses and which of the following? (*select all that apply*)

1. Educational materials
2. Support groups
3. Statistics on incidence of disease
4. Data on exacerbations
5. Sibling support
6. Hospice information

SAFETY *STAT!*

Short Answer Question

Describe five concerns a pediatric nurse should be assessing for when caring for a child with chronic illness experiencing an exacerbation of symptoms or an acute phase of the illness.

1. _____

2. _____

3. _____

4. _____

5. _____

SAFETY *STAT!*

Fill-in-the-Blank Question

A child with a chronic illness is at risk for experiencing many symptoms associated with their illness. Especially during periods of an acute exacerbation, the child is in need for symptom control. Symptom control and management is the pediatric nurse's responsibility. Seven symptoms a child with a

chronic illness is at risk for include _____, _____,

_____, _____, _____,

_____, and _____.

PATIENT TEACHING GUIDELINES

Short Answer Question

The father of a child with a chronic illness asks about how best to handle the child's emotions, outbursts, and frustrations. The nurse would be correct in providing information about expectations of behavior for the child. List three topics the nurse can discuss with the father:

1. _____

2. _____

3. _____

TEAM WORKS

Fill-in-the-Blank Question

A child with a complicated chronic illness who is now experiencing the end of life is showing progression toward death. The physiological responses to death can produce common symptoms of impending death that include the following six clinical signs:

_____, _____, _____,

_____, _____, and _____.

Legal Aspects of Pediatric Nursing Care

Name: _____

Date: _____

Course: _____

Instructor: _____

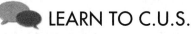 LEARN TO C.U.S.

Short Answer Questions

1. A fellow nurse has asked you to co-sign the medication administration record for a patient who is severely cognitively impaired, in postoperative surgical discomfort, and requiring narcotic medications for pain. The nurse explains that she needed to give the maximum amount of morphine intravenously for this patient, who was demonstrating a high level of pain behaviors. You did not see the nurse get the medication out of the computerized medication administration machine, count the remaining number of morphine vials, double-check the dose in the syringe, or watch her waste the remaining drug not used. What is your best response?

_____

_____

_____

_____

_____

2. A physician has entered an order into the electronic medical health record for a dose of lorazepam (Ativan®) PO to be given to a child who is experiencing breakthrough nausea in the immediate post-operative period. The dose ordered is considered out of range for the child's weight and you are uncomfortable giving the medication when you calculate a dose amount that should be lower. What is the best way to approach the situation? Whom do you call and how can you phrase your concern?

_____

_____

_____

_____

_____

THERAPEUTIC COMMUNICATION

Fill-in-the-Blank Question

1. A nurse is responsible for maintaining HIPAA, which stands for _____

_____ _____ and _____

_____.

Short Answer Question

2. The nurse should explain to a family friend who is calling on the telephone to get an update on a child's condition that HIPAA prevents the nurse from giving out health information. How can the nurse explain this to the family friend and what should the nurse ask the family friend to do?

_____

_____

_____

TEAM WORKS

Short Answer Question

Describe the process of reporting a concern about a colleague that you suspect is having personal issues with drugs. You have been concerned by certain behaviors that have caused you to suspect substance abuse and impaired clinical practice or clinical judgment.

_____

_____

_____

_____

_____

PATIENT TEACHING GUIDELINES

Short Answer Questions

1. You have been asked by a hospitalized child's father to provide the phone number of an administrator so that he can make a complaint about the care provided by the pediatric health-care team. How do you handle this situation?

_____

_____

_____

2. A mother of a child newly diagnosed with acute lymphocytic leukemia notices that another family on the floor has a similarly aged child with alopecia. The mother calls you in and asks you whether the child also has cancer and is there for cancer treatment, and whether or not she can meet the child's mother to learn more about the family's experience with childhood cancer. What are your next steps?

_____

_____

_____

CONCEPTUAL CORNERSTONE

Short Answer Questions

Define each of the concepts below and describe how each concept relates to legal aspects of pediatric health care. Then give one example of an issue that would fall under these concepts.

Legal aspects of care

Definition: _____

Related issue: _____

Safety

Definition: _____

Related issue: _____

Communication

Definition: _____

Related issue: _____

Professionalism

Definition: _____

Related issue: _____

TRUE OR FALSE QUESTION

_____ Nurses who perform CPR in the community on a child who suffers an accident and requires resuscitation efforts will always be covered by the Good Samaritan Act.

FILL-IN-THE-BLANK QUESTION

The _____ is a nonprofit organization whose purpose is to provide an umbrella organization for all individual State Boards of Nursing. This organization provides a mechanism for communication, counsel, and the development of standards for issues concerning the safety and welfare of public health.

Providing a Safe Environment: Home and School

6

Name: _____

Date: _____

Course: _____

Instructor: _____

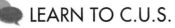 LEARN TO C.U.S.

Short Answer Question

The nurse caring for a newborn on the pediatric unit was observing the teen mother in her handling of her infant. The newborn was born at a local hospital, was considered full-term at 38 weeks gestation, and was discharged home after an uncomplicated birthing experience. The baby was checked during the first pediatrician's well infant follow-up appointment and was found to be significantly hyperbilirubinemic with a serum level of 14.8. The newborn was admitted to the pediatric unit for phototherapy and observation. The pediatric nurse became quite concerned when he witnessed the new mother pulling the infant down to the end of the isolette by the ankle, and not supporting the infant's head when she picked up the infant to feed him. How might the nurse use the C.U.S. method to communicate his concerns?

C: _____

U: _____

S: _____

CONCEPTUAL CORNERSTONE: SAFETY

Short Answer Questions

1. Define the concept of safety as it relates to an infant's first year of life.

_____

_____

2. Describe four general categories of areas of safety concerns for an infant:

_____

_____

_____

_____

TEAM WORKS

Short Answer Question

Who is responsible for providing safety to children across the developmental period? (*List no less than 10*)

1. _____

2. _____

3. _____

4. _____

5. _____

6. _____

7. _____

8. _____

9. _____

10. _____

SAFETY *STAT!*

Review Questions

1. Pacifiers are often used to provide both an opportunity for a young infant to suck, as well as to provide comfort. Parents need specific guidelines on how to select safe pacifiers. Which of the following is the highest priority in selecting a pacifier for a young infant?
   1. One that is dishwasher safe as the pacifier needs the high temperatures for sterilization
   2. One that is the right size for the infant's mouth
   3. One that has a finger ring for quick removal
   4. One that is made from one single piece of synthetic material

2. Older infants are becoming more mobile and place everything in their mouths that they can pick up. Older infants have an increased risk for poisoning. The following list gives poisons considered the most dangerous except:
   1. Antifreeze
   2. Oven cleaners
   3. Fuels, such as gasoline and kerosene
   4. Cosmetics, such as deodorant

3. While working in a public health clinic, a family states that they are concerned about the safety of their children, because they could not afford to pay for the gas bill to heat their home and have resorted to using a small outdoor cooking device for heat. Your best answer to the concern of carbon monoxide poisoning with this type of indoor heating device is to say which of the following:
   1. Carbon monoxide can kill but it takes several exposures to the toxic substance.
   2. As long as adequate ventilation is provided, this type of heating device is safe.
   3. Carbon monoxide is colorless and tasteless but has a strong odor so is easily identifiable.
   4. This type of heating is not safe for indoor use and has fatal toxic effects.

4. Infant and toddler cribs should be used with safety bars or slats. If the space between the crib bars or slats is more than _____ inches apart, an infant can get a limb or their neck stuck or wedged, and suffer injuries or death.
   1. 2 and 3/8
   2. 2 and 5/8
   3. 3 and 3/8
   4. 3 and 5/8

SAFETY *STAT!*

True or False Questions

1. _____ The only approved means to leaving an older infant or young toddler in a bath alone for a few moments is to prop the young child into a federally-approved plastic bath seat with a secure rim.

2. _____ Ipecac syrup is an over-the-counter medication known to induce vomiting related to toxic ingestion; it is used readily in emergency settings as it works with activated charcoal and whole-bowel irrigation for the removal of toxic ingestions.

CONCEPTUAL CORNERSTONE
Matching Exercise

Match the definition with the corresponding key term.

1. Near-drowning
2. Toxicology
3. Ipecac syrup

A. An over-the-counter medication known to induce vomiting related to toxic ingestion; it is no longer used in health-care settings as it has been replaced with activated charcoal and whole-bowel irrigation.

B. A liquid substance used to induce vomiting. Only obtainable by a prescription, this medication must be kept locked and safe from children as it has a sweet flavor.

C. A phrase used to denote a level of survival after an immersion in water.

D. The study of harmful or poisonous levels of chemicals in the body, including their detection, avoidance, chemistry, pharmacological actions, antidotes, and treatments.

E. A section of the science of forensic medicine, this is the study of what caused morbidity (causes of illness) and mortality (causes of death) in children.

TEAM WORKS: SAFETY ON THE HOSPITAL UNIT
Short Answer Question

List 10 components of a pediatric unit safety check.

1. _____
2. _____
3. _____
4. _____
5. _____
6. _____
7. _____
8. _____
9. _____
10. _____

CULTURAL CONSIDERATIONS: CULTURE AND PERSPECTIVES ABOUT SAFETY

Short Answer Question

Define co-sleeping and describe the safety risks associated:

_____

_____

_____

_____

_____

_____

_____

PATIENT TEACHING GUIDELINES: SAFETY IN BULLYING SITUATIONS

True or False Questions

1. _____ Only associated with male adolescents, bullying has been associated with self-mutilation, depression, and suicide.

2. _____ Although not addressed by school district offices, anti-bullying policies are developed by teachers to protect students within the classroom setting.

3. _____ School-age bullying is typically not associated with sexual identification, gender, or ethnicity.

DRUG FACTS

Review Question

A child is being seen in the pediatric clinic for a single dog-bite wound. The wound is to be irrigated prior to the pediatrician suturing the wound closed. The most appropriate solution to irrigate a dog-bite wound is which of the following:
1. Dextrose 5% with 0.9% normal saline
2. 0.45% normal saline
3. 5% povidone-iodine
4. 1% povidone-iodine

Families Experiencing Stressors

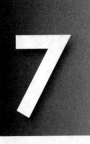

Name: _____

Date: _____

Course: _____

Instructor: _____

💬 THERAPEUTIC COMMUNICATION

True or False Questions

1. _____ Emergency departments and critical or intensive care units are the two most common areas for pediatric nurses to see families in stress.

2. _____ The definition of a mediating process is when two groups get together to make a plan for the child's care in order to reduce stress felt by all.

CONCEPTUAL CORNERSTONE

Short Answer Question

Coping is a concept that describes a person's adaptation to a perceived stressor or stressful event. How might positive and negative coping be identified?

   Positive coping behaviors:

   _____

   _____

   _____

   Negative coping behaviors:

   _____

   _____

   _____

TEAM WORKS

Short Answer Questions

1. According to Selye's theory on stress and coping, when stress occurs, it activates a series of neurologic and hormonal processes within the brain and body systems. The duration and intensity of stress can cause short-term or long-term effects. If adaptation does not occur, disease processes may result. What is the title of the process that the body goes through when exposed to stress, and when the body activates a serious of neurological and hormonal processes?

_____

2. Define the following three terms:

   1. Pediatric Medical Traumatic Stress (PMTS): _____

   2. Post-Traumatic Stress Syndrome: _____

   3. Post-Traumatic Stress Disorder: _____

True or False Questions

1. _____ High levels of stress are always apparent to see in a parent of a child suffering from a significant injury and will present as both physical and psychological symptoms.

2. _____ It is estimated that every year 25% of children sustain an unintentional injury or illness that requires medical care or hospitalization, and ~ 50% of emergency department visits are pediatric patients.

3. _____ Spiritual distress is only seen in those who are practicing in a particular faith and/or who belong to a religious institution.

4. _____ The pediatric health-care team can assist a family member who is experiencing spiritual distress during a child's serious condition or during a lengthy hospitalization by understanding the characteristics of this type of distress. Characteristics of spiritual distress include contemplating questions pertaining to life, death, purpose, suffering, inner peace, love, attachment, despair, a higher being, alienation, and religion.

PATIENT TEACHING GUIDELINES

Short Answer Question

List 10 stress-reducing behaviors that a pediatric nurse can offer as guidelines to assist a family when their child is hospitalized.

1. _____

2. _____

3. _____

4. _____

5. _____

6. _____

7. _____

8. _____

9. _____

10. _____

CULTURAL CONSIDERATIONS

Short Answer Question

A family of a child who has been admitted after a motor vehicle accident that caused a significant head injury and multiple fractures is waiting in the family room outside of the pediatric intensive care unit. Many family members are sitting by themselves, quietly. There is very little apparent interaction and no one has asked to speak to a team member about the status of the child.

1. How might you interpret this behavior?
2. Are there cultural threads here that might be important to note while deciding how best to help the family cope with the stressful situation?

SAFETY *STAT!*

True or False Question

_____ Stress can be difficult to define as many consider the experience of stress as a unique and sub-jective experience. *Stress* is often defined as a state of being after a perceived threat or un-due demand has taken place, or a significant change in the environment has taken place, that can be perceived as damaging, or be actually damaging to one's physiological being.

Short Answer Question

During a team conference at a public health clinic, the pediatrician and pediatric nurse practitioner share the most common reasons that children are admitted to an acute care hospital. List the top seven reasons for these hospital admissions:

1. _____

2. _____

3. _____

4. _____

5. _____

6. _____

7. _____

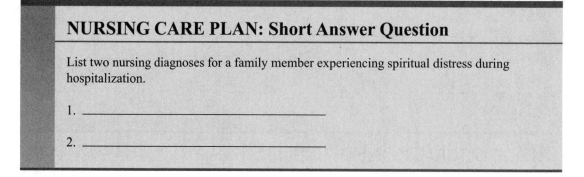

NURSING CARE PLAN: Short Answer Question

List two nursing diagnoses for a family member experiencing spiritual distress during hospitalization.

1. _____

2. _____

HEALTH PROMOTION

Review Question

Working in a position as a home care pediatric nurse, you notice that the family's level of stress is increasing. Your concerns for both short-term and long-term consequences of stress are increasing. Long-term consequences of post-traumatic stress syndrome include which of the following:

1. Long-term functional impairment

2. Increased divorce rates

3. Increased sibling suicides

4. Frequent illness in the home